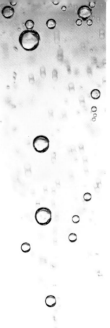

BALANCING SENSES
THE SIX SENSES SPA BOOK

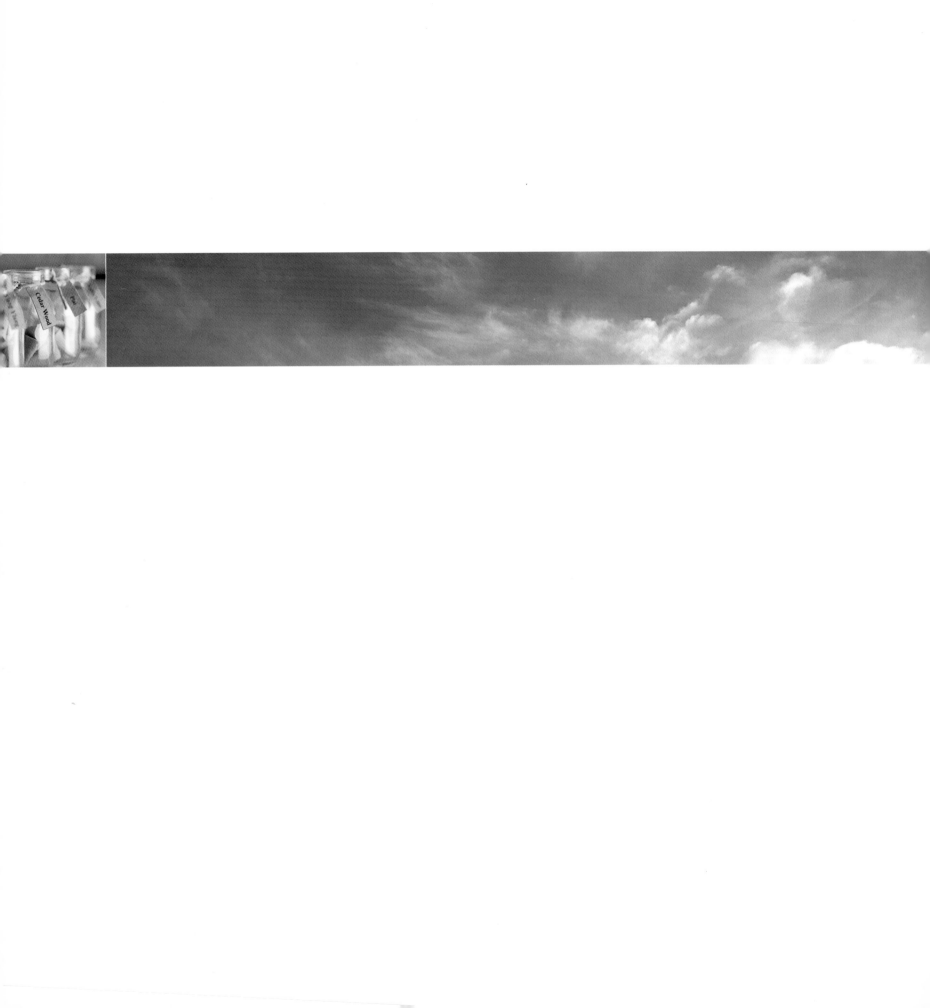

BALANCING SENSES

THE SIX SENSES
SPA BOOK

KATE O'BRIEN / Text
JÖRG SUNDERMANN / Photography

Editions Didier Millet

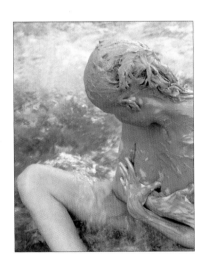

Mineral rich mud helps draw impurities leaving the skin cleansed and smooth. OPPOSITE: The outdoor pool at Six Senses Spa in Bodrum, Turkey looks out over the sparkling Aegean Sea.

Executive Editor
MELISA TEO

Senior Editor
JOANNA GREENFIELD

Designer
CHAN HUI YEE

Production Manager
SIN KAM CHEONG

Photography Director
MELISA TEO

Photographer's Assistants
KEITH MILLER / CHERYL FAN /
COLLIN PATRICK / JONATHAN ANG

Project Director for Six Senses
RAYMOND HALL

Chef
REMON ALPHENAAR

SIX SENSES RESORTS & SPAS
19/F Two Pacific Place
142 Sukhumvit Road
Bangkok 10110, Thailand
www.sixsenses.com

First published in 2007 by
EDITIONS DIDIER MILLET PTE LTD
121 Telok Ayer Street
#03-01, Singapore 068590
www.edmbooks.com

Photography © Six Senses Resorts & Spa
© 2007 Editions Didier Millet Pte Ltd

Printed in Singapore.

ISBN 10: 981-4155-84-5
ISBN 13: 978-981-4155-84-7

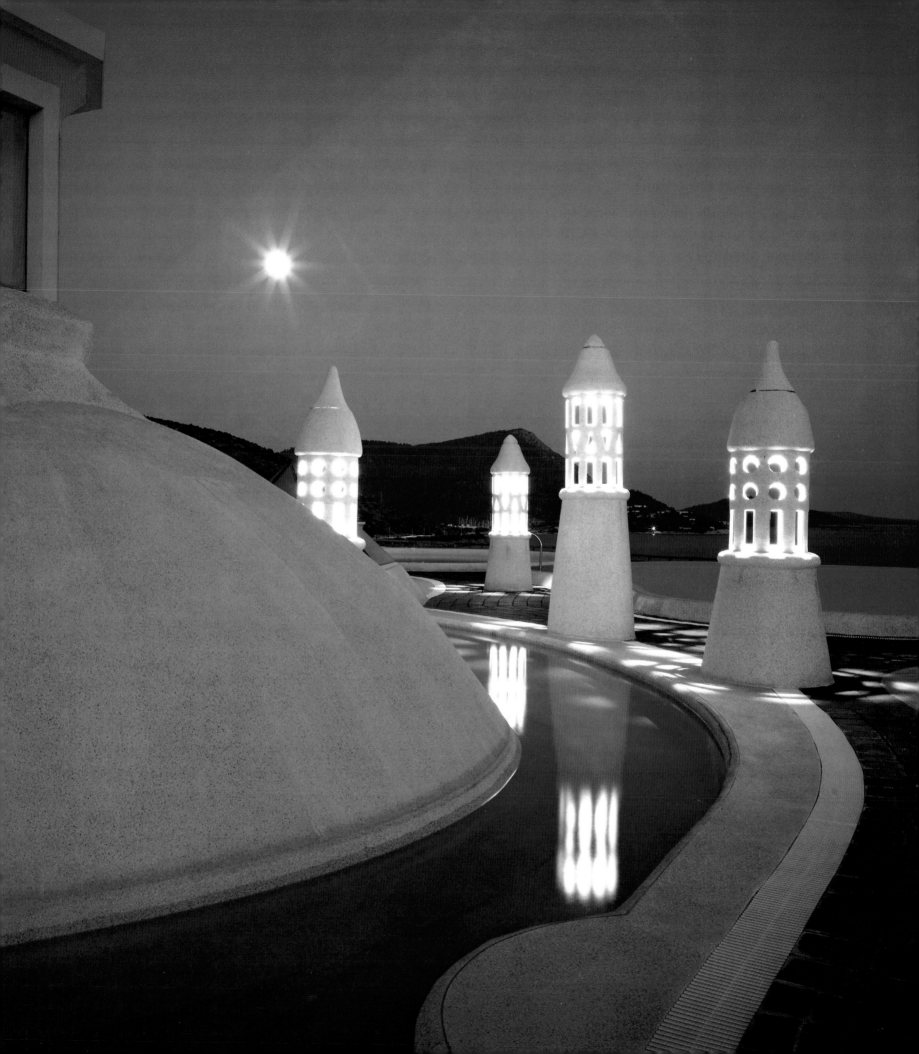

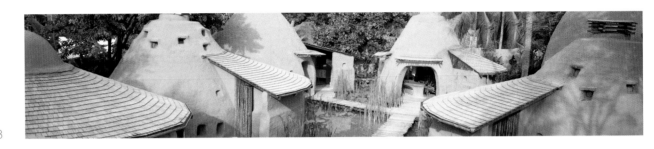
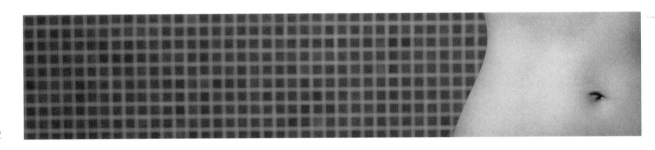
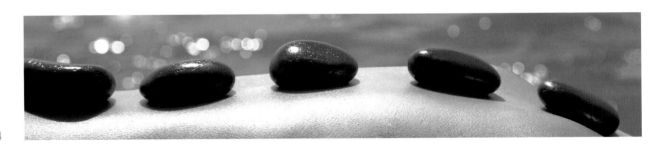

CONTENTS

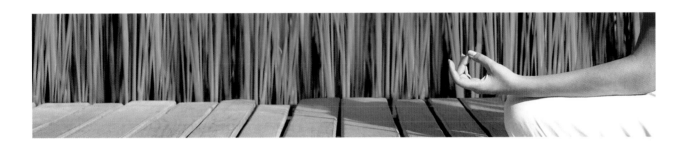

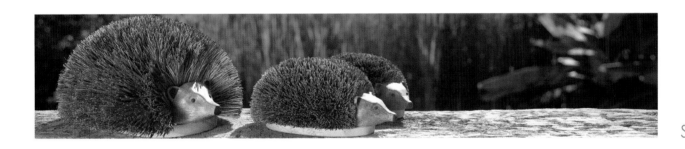

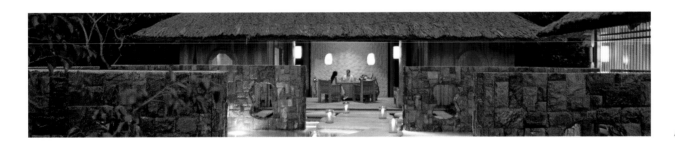

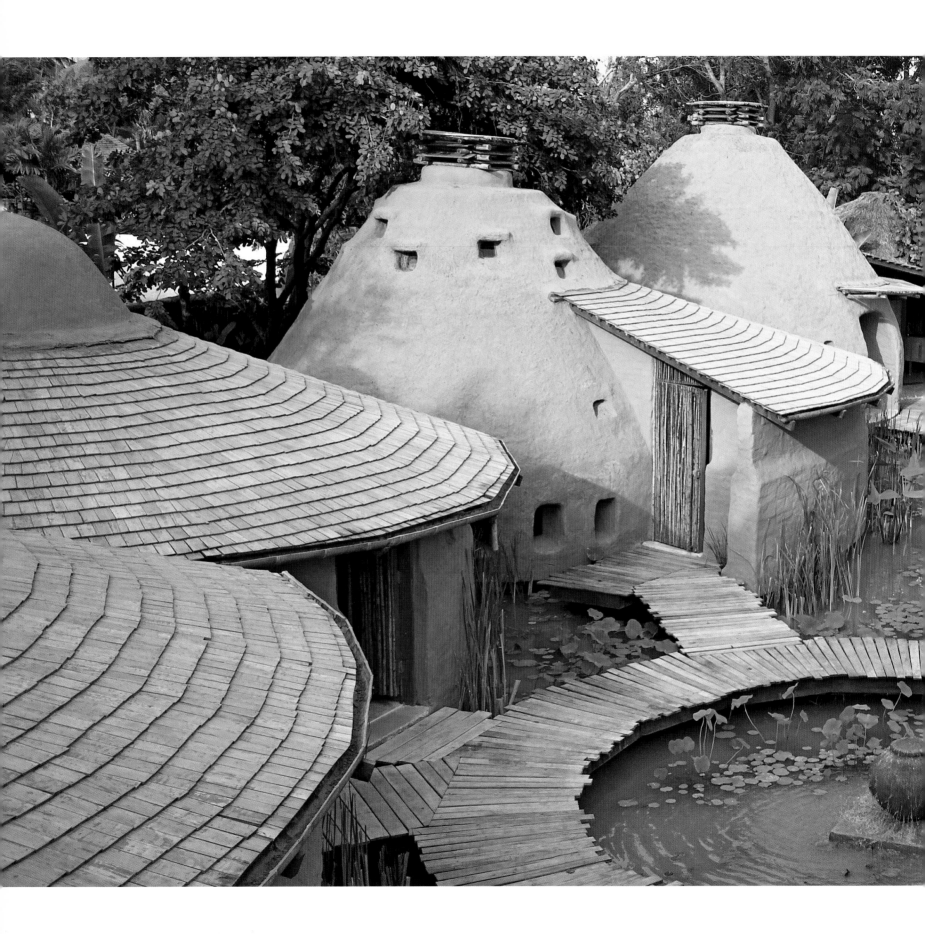

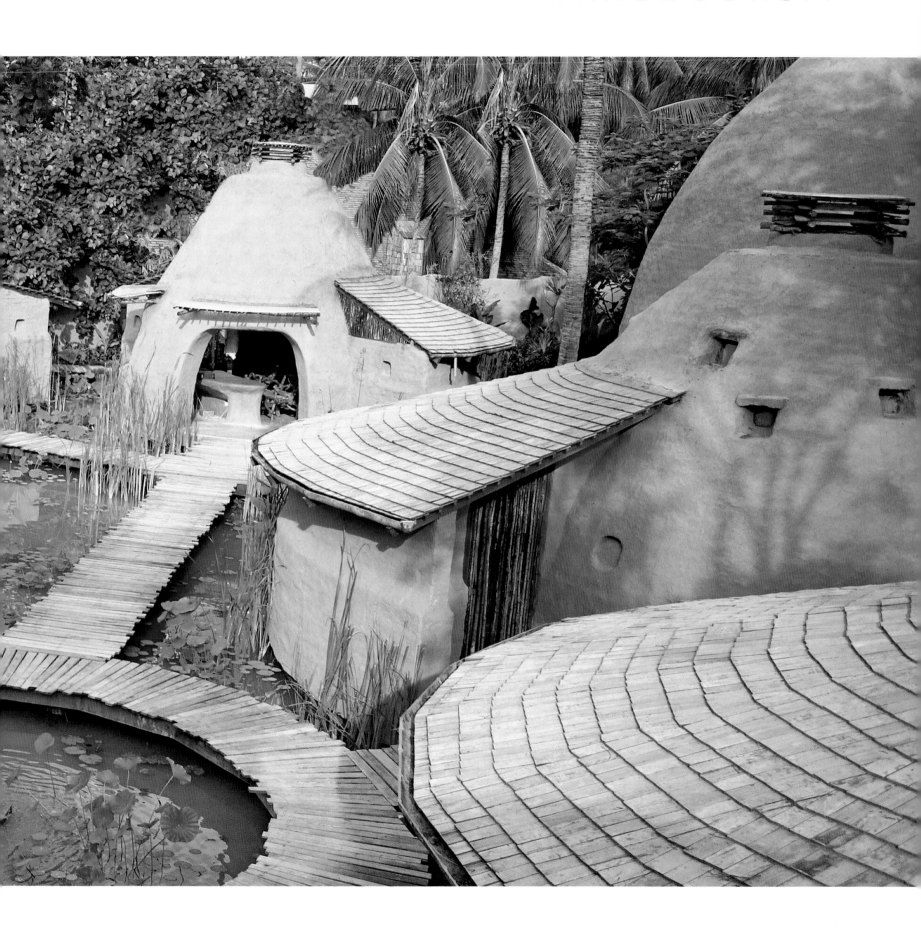

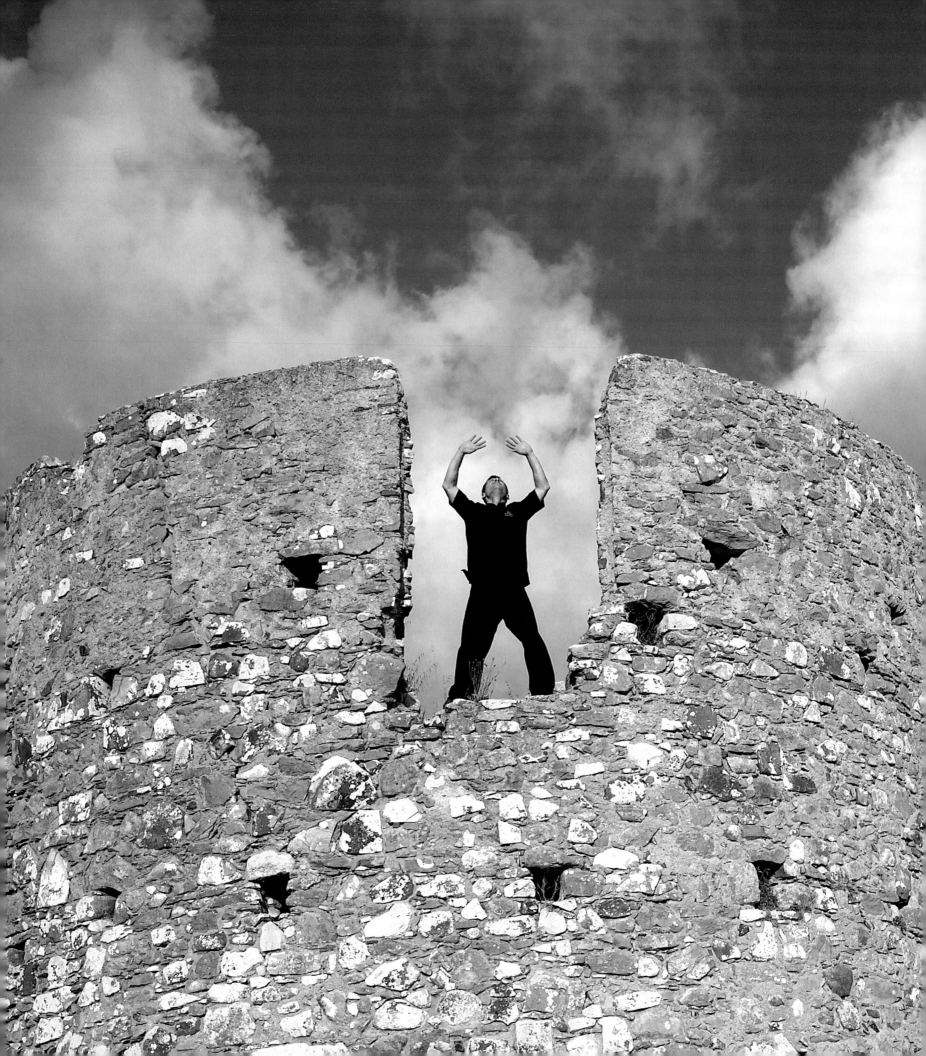

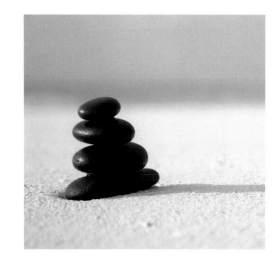

BALANCING SENSES

Balancing Senses is a fresh and truly holistic approach to life. Created by Six Senses, an industry leader in well-being, this essential and authoritative guide helps you make the most of what you were born with and live and be as you were born to.

Supported by ancient time-honoured healing secrets from India and China, *Balancing Senses* offers an insight into how these ancient healing philosophies combine so perfectly with modern scientific knowledge about how the body works. Packed with easy-to-master recipes for nurturing both body and spirit fashioned by Six Senses leading chefs, the concept of *Balancing Senses* will help keep you looking and feeling your best for always.

If losing weight or boosting energy is the aim, then *Body Sense* will help you on your way to health and vitality. Overflowing with colourful platters of supernutrient-rich, herb-enlivened sumptuous foods, packed with all things good and nourishing, detoxing couldn't be easier. There are easy-to-follow, mouth-watering recipes and pertinent body care advice to help you look and feel younger, fitter and stronger. Even better, these recipes will set the whole family on the way to long-term health.

Beauty Sense is packed with tips on holding back the hands of time with simple, age-defying, recipes to nourish the skin, hair and nails and guides you to vibrant, glowing skin inside and out.

Lives today are busier than ever with more things to do and more goals to achieve. In spite of this, many of us are fast losing sight of who we really are. We all have the answers within; it's simply a matter of listening to them and acting on what they tell us. By working with age-old spiritually uplifting therapies such as yoga, t'ai chi, pranayama and meditation, *Mind Sense* addresses this need and takes you on a healing journey towards a heightened sense of well-being. As more and more Western medical practitioners embrace the world of wellness, they too appreciate that listening to the voice within may be the answer to many of today's health crises. This is preventive medicine at its best and the heart of ayurvedic and traditional Chinese medicine (TCM) philosophies.

We can't alter genetics but we can capitalize on what we have by taking a little more time for ourselves. *Balancing Senses* is no fad diet. It's a way of living. All you need is time and willingness to immerse yourself into this programme of positive change and, most of all, to enjoy every moment of it.

Namaste.

Basalt stones, whether hot or cold, are a common sight in today's spas. Used to revitalize the body's energy points, the stones help restore inner balance.
OPPOSITE: T'ai chi and *qi gong* will help the body find its inner rhythm, ensuring balance and harmony.

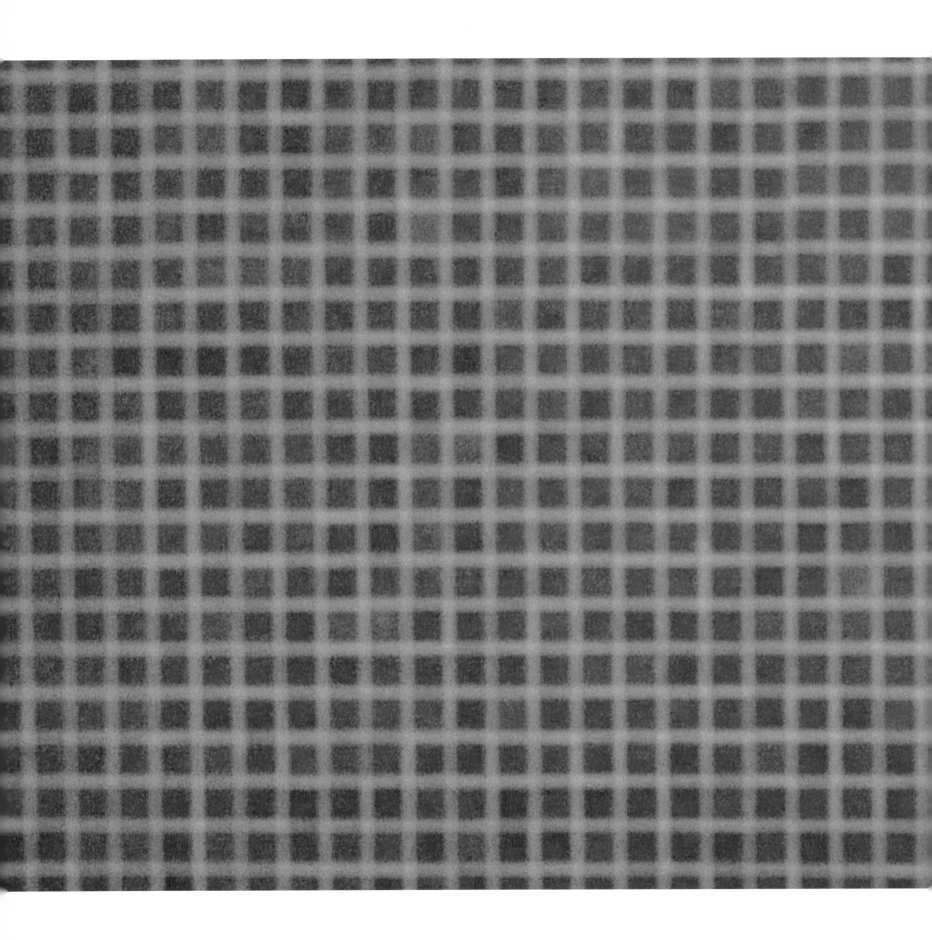

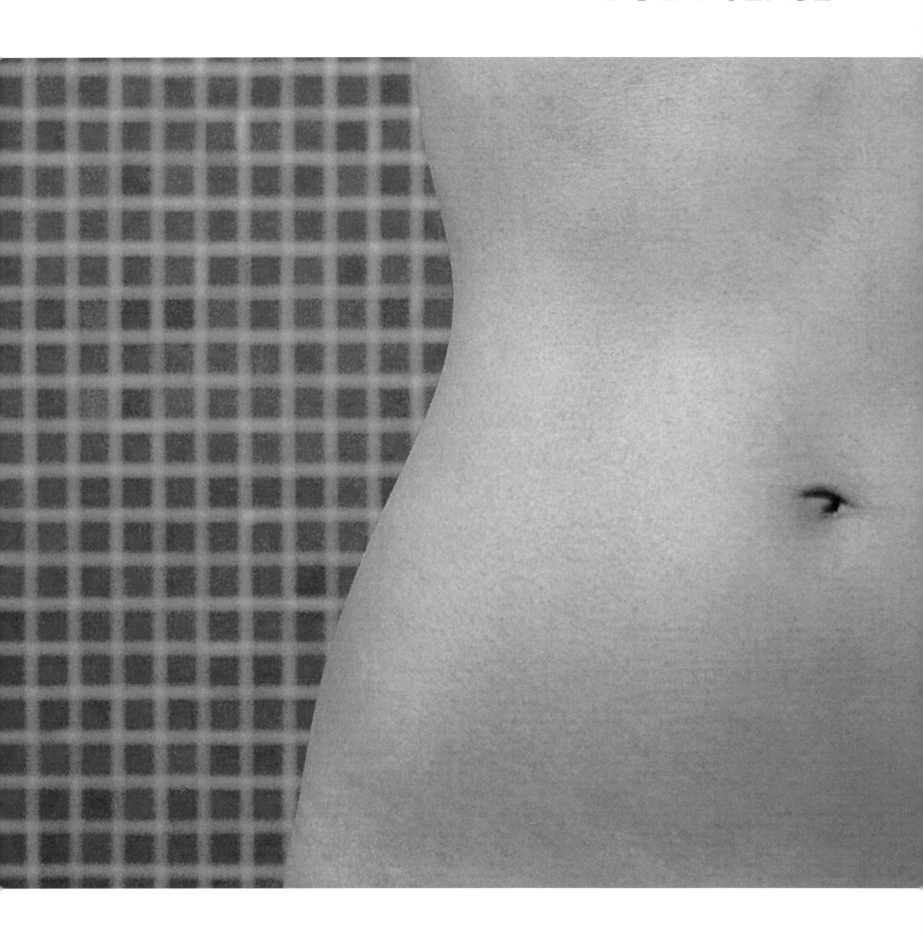

BODY SENSE

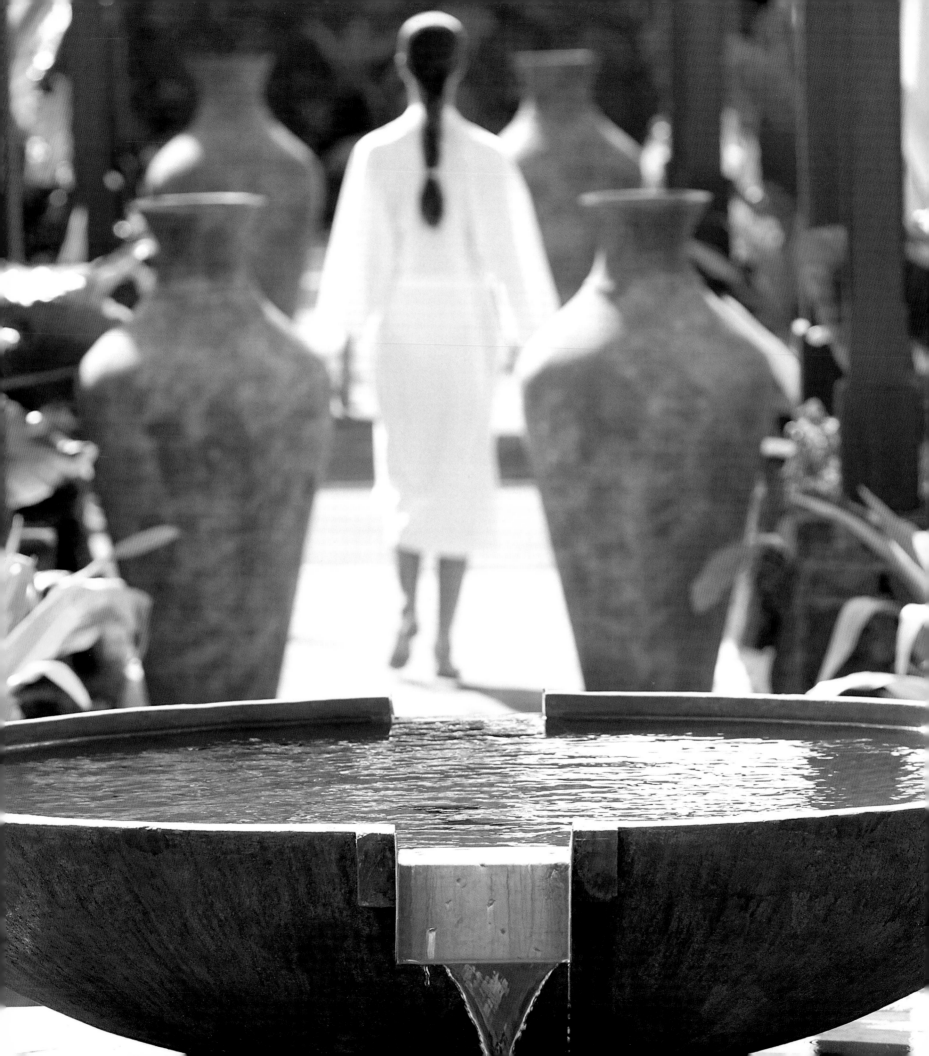

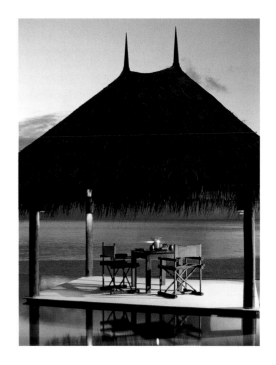

BODY SENSE
Be the change you want to see.

-Mahatma Gandhi

In recent years, the original interpretation of spa cuisine has gone from the glorified health farm style of regimented bland eating to simply delicious meals packed with organic, fresh, wholesome and seasonal foods to help you make the most of you. This latter cuisine is what *Balancing Senses* is all about and if a healthy toned body, radiant skin and hair, amazing vitality and a strong mind are what you are after, then here are the answers.

Focusing on your health from inside with energizing, colourful and wholesome foods, *Body Sense* is based upon trusted and time-honoured ayurvedic and traditional Chinese medicine (TCM) principles combined with the cutting-edge rationale of the glycaemic index that promises not just a slimmer body but also radiant skin and a strong, stable and centred mind. This fresh approach to eating is easy to apply in the home when cooking for the whole family, with super nutrient-packed and easy-to-follow recipes which will leave you lighter, calmer and completely energized.

As science evolves, we are learning that it is not just a particular nutrient that is beneficial to health but the whole food. Consequently there is less emphasis on eating specific foods rich in a particular vitamin or mineral and more on the nutritional benefits of the whole food or meal. Healthy eating today is less about denial and more about eating vital and colourful foods that help maintain health and fight disease. Think juices overflowing with super foods, colourful platters of lightly cooked vegetables enlivened with herbs and spices, tender pieces of tuna or salmon each brimming with vitamins and minerals that nourish the body from the inside. With not an E-number or factory-farmed animal in sight, detoxing has never been easier. What's more, food loaded with natural flavour does not need extra seasoning, so salt is replaced with tastier herbal alternatives.

Everyone knows that there is more to food than it being good for you; for the sophisticated palate it must look and taste great too. Rest assured, it does. Each page is overflowing with tips to help you on your road to better health by becoming more shopping savvy when it comes to buying food, knowing what to look out for when choosing vegetables, fish or olive oil and the know-how you need to set yourself on the way to maximizing flavour and goodness when you cook.

Enjoy some peace and tranquillity at Soneva Gili, as you dine at your own private over-water sala. OPPOSITE: Taking time for yourself and treating your body with care will ensure you feel good about how you look and content with the person within.

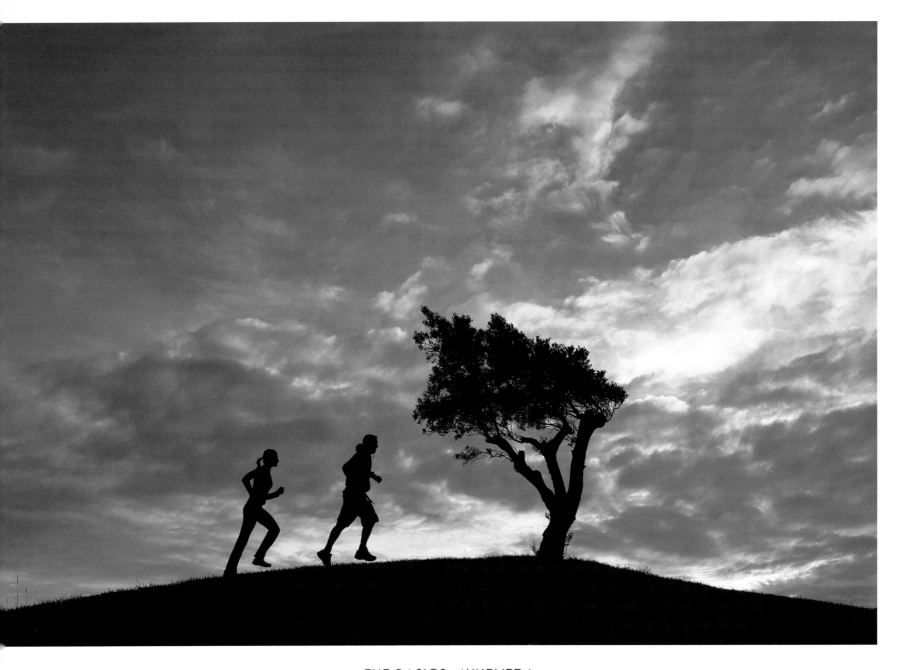

The ancient philosophers believed that living and working with nature keep both body and mind in balance and harmony. OPPOSITE (FROM TOP): Fresh leaves infused with a light and tasty dressing make ideal summer food; Colourful fresh juices are deliciously light and nutritious.

THE BASICS: AYURVEDA Translated from the ancient Indian language of Sanskrit, ayurveda literally means the science of life and is regarded by scholars as the oldest healing system in the world. It remains to this day the prime healing tradition adopted by the people of India, Sri Lanka and Nepal. Furthermore—thanks to the prolific teachings of holistic lifestyle guru Deepak Chopra and a host of celebrity devotees—the secrets of this ancient discipline are as popular and as widely used now as ever before.

At the heart of ayurvedic philosophy is the concept that our bodies are a microcosm of the universe with three universal forces at work: *vata* (air), *pitta* (fire) and *kapha* (earth). These are called *doshas*, and just as each of us has an individual face or thumbprint, we also have a unique pattern of energy that corresponds with these *doshas*. This combination of our physical, mental and emotional characteristics is our inherent constitution. Achieving balance and harmony between the *doshas* is the foundation of health and well-being in ayurvedic medicine. While one *dosha* is generally dominant, ayurveda believes that all individuals possess *vata*, *pitta* and *kapha* in varying degrees. (See box on page 18.)

We are said to be in good health when the *doshas* are balanced and, to achieve this, ayurveda treats the body, mind and spirit as a unified entity in order to maintain this inner balance and harmony.

A quick test to determine your dominant *dosha* is to ask yourself how you usually handle stress. If you feel nervous and anxious, you are probably of *vata* temperament. Impatience and anger are hot-tempered *pitta* characteristics, while *kapha* types often feel uninspired, depressed and lethargic.

As ayurvedic medicine is founded on the belief that all disease stems from the digestive system, food is a central component of ayurvedic philosophy and should be enjoyed for health and longevity. While different foods may be recommended for specific constitutional imbalances, the overall emphasis lies very much on unprocessed, fresh and seasonal foods to energize the body and prevent toxic build-up.

GUIDELINES FOR BALANCED AYURVEDIC EATING

- Aim to eat at a similar time each day, preferably to coincide with the sun's energy. Ideally, breakfast should be taken around sunrise, lunch about noon, when the sun is at its highest point, and dinner ideally by sunset, but no later than 7.30 pm.
- Eat calmly and slowly and enjoy your food without outside distraction, such as television.
- As appetite and digestive function vary with the seasons, food should be chosen

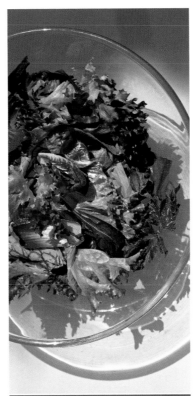

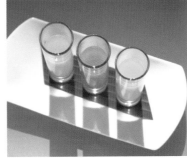

according to the season, your individual constitution and any specific *dosha* imbalances. For example, spring is *kapha*, meaning less food is needed than in winter. Summer is *pitta* with increased need for cooling food and, as the digestive system increases during the *vata* period of autumn and winter, heavier, warmer and well-cooked food is recommended as it is more easily digested.

- Foods are generally divided into heavy, such as potatoes, bread and rice, and light, vegetables and juices, with emphasis on heavy food during the earlier part of the day and on lighter food in the evening.
- Raw food should not be eaten at the same time as cooked.
- Fruit should be eaten seasonally and on its own.
- Drink plenty of fluids during the day. Drink small sips of water with meals.
- Use lots of fresh herbs and spices when cooking, especially those associated with the individual *doshas*.

WHY MAKE BODY SENSE PART OF YOUR LIFE?

Firstly and most importantly, *Body Sense* will help you look and feel strong.

Eating foods packed with nutrients and skin-saving antioxidant properties will help your body fight disease.

Rather than a restrictive regime, *Body Sense* means you can have fabulous-tasting food and never feel deprived.

Body Sense allows you to eat normal food that's ideal for all the family.

Lastly, it really works. This is not a fad diet, but a realistic lifestyle.

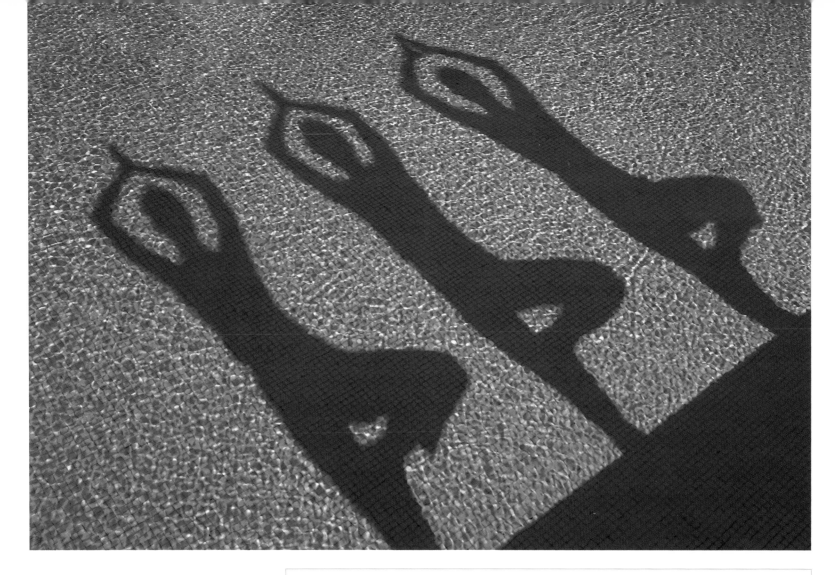

The ancient Masters say that yoga *asanas*, such as the tree pose, build strength and stability in the body. OPPOSITE (FROM TOP): Water is essential to the body; The symbol of yin and yang, a central tenet of TCM.

	VATA	PITTA	KAPHA
CHARACTERISTIC	Dry	Hot	Stable
PHYSICAL MAKE-UP	Small boned and light.	Medium bone structure.	Strong boned and prone to weight gain.
DISPOSITION	Friendly, social, fast learner, artistic. Fast eater, prone to constipation.	Ambitious, passionate, hot tempered, intelligent, exudes wisdom. Generally eats sensibly with a tendency towards diarrhoea.	Earth mother, loving, truthful, resourceful, nurtures and provides. Enjoys food and eating.
APPETITE	Variable appetite and digestion. Should eat warm cooked food and sweet, sour, salty tastes to balance. Should avoid fried food.	Strong metabolism and good digestion. Should eat sweet, bitter and astringent tastes to balance and choose more cool and raw food.	Slow, steady appetite with efficient digestion. Responds best to warm and cooked food.
SKIN TYPE	Tendency towards dry skin and fine lines.	Normal to combination skin with tendency towards oiliness.	Skin can be oily.
SEASON	Autumn/Winter	Summer	Spring

THE BASICS: TRADITIONAL CHINESE MEDICINE

With the present shift from Western thinking to a more integrative mind and body approach, Taoism, the fundamental philosophy of the world's oldest civilization, is as relevant today as it was in classical China. With the emphasis firmly on diet, movement, spiritual and emotional well-being, TCM treats the body as a whole and aims to prevent illness by maintaining overall health and balance.

In Taoist belief, the universe exists as a unified whole, comprising two opposing yet complementary forces known as yin and yang. It is the dynamics between these forces that govern *qi*, the vital energy that powers the universe and suffuses every living cell.

When a person is in good health the movement of *qi* and blood through the body is harmonious. However, if *qi* or blood is blocked or slowed, the organs, tissues and cells will be deprived of the power needed to function at their best. Traditional Chinese therapies like acupuncture, moxabustion, acupressure, reflexology and exercise routines, such as *qi gong* and t'ai chi, work towards removing blockages and encouraging a smoother flow of *qi* around the whole body.

Although each of us is an individual, Chinese medicine maintains that regardless of make-up we must maintain overall harmony with the natural world by matching nature's cycles and eating with the seasons. Root vegetables, being warming, are more plentiful during the colder winter months, while summer is the time for light, clean food with abundant supplies of cooling fresh fruits and leafy greens. Even in tropical climates where heat is constant, food should be primarily light and lean with the emphasis on fresh leafy greens, fruits, leaner meats and fish, with less dairy products and refined carbohydrates. Skipping meals is not encouraged, nor is eating large meals late in the evening, which results in indigestion, stomach discomfort and fitful sleep. By simply eating earlier, 2–3 hours before bed, and eating less—follow the 75 per cent rule where the stomach is half full with food, one quarter with liquid and one quarter empty—sluggishness will disappear and health and sleep patterns will improve.

Water is essential, especially in hotter climates, but forcing eight glasses of water into the body can be as detrimental as not drinking any. Listen to your body. In warmer climates, cooling drinks like grape or watermelon juice, green tea and water are good, while cooler weather dictates more warming fluids.

Consult a qualified physician before starting an ayurvedic or TCM programme.

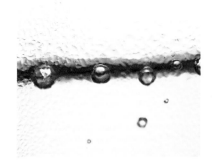

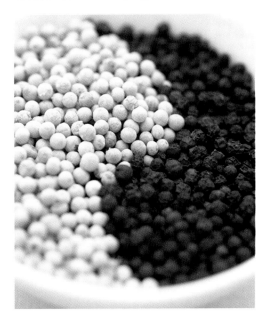

SLOW FOOD

The idea of slow food links the pleasure of eating with awareness and responsibility, meaning that the enjoyment of excellent food and wine should be combined with efforts to save traditional food such as cheese, grains, vegetables, fruit, and animal breeds that are disappearing due to the prevalence of convenient fast food. The Slow Food Organization seeks to protect invaluable food heritage in a world where the pleasures of taste are not always learned through leisurely meals eaten around a lively table and through its understanding of gastronomy, agriculture and the environment. The movement has become an active player in agriculture and ecology.

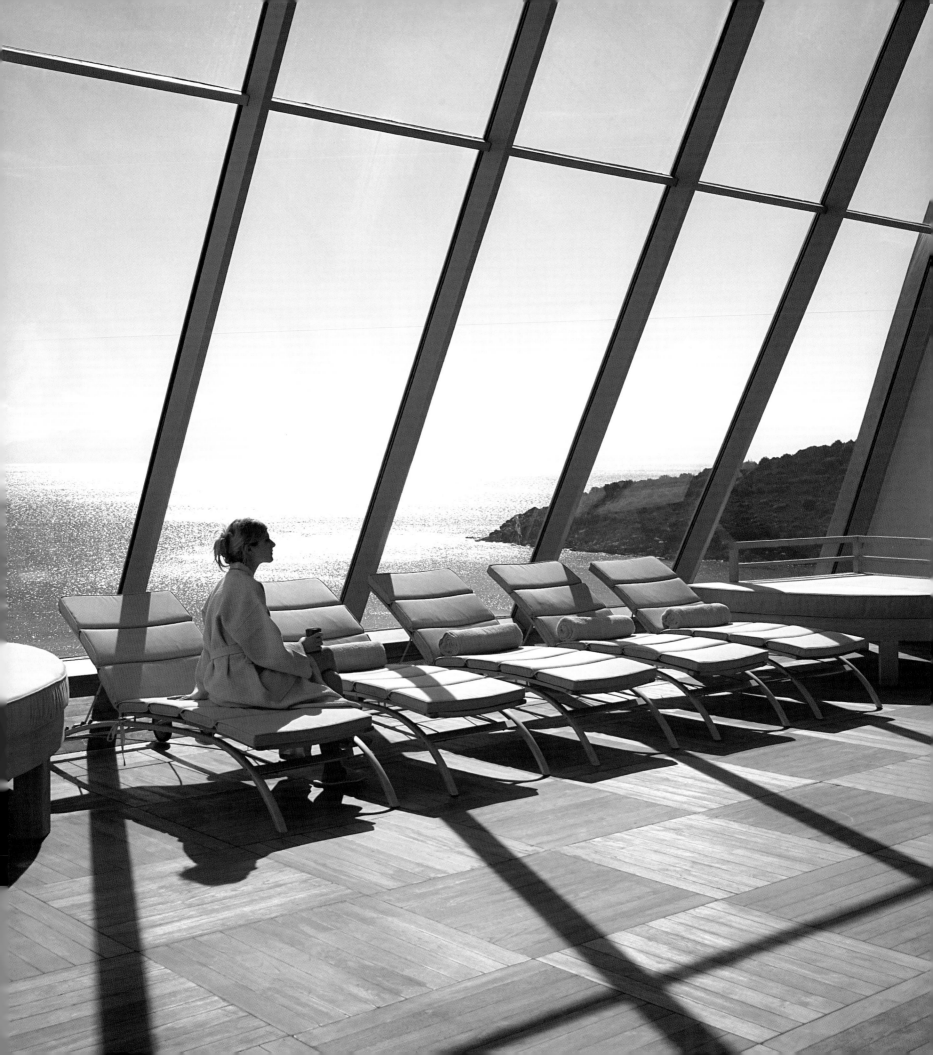

BOOSTING ENERGY NATURALLY

We spend time, money and energy itself in the quest for a renewed and energized body. Energy, the greatest life force, depends on us getting clean air, sleep, water and eating as close to nature as possible so the sun, air and water can flow unimpeded through our work, exercise and emotional expression. However, for the majority of us, running on empty and waking up feeling exhausted has become the norm. Living the *Balancing Senses* way gives you everything your body needs to keep it charged through the day and beyond. Hunger pangs will for the most part be forgotten and, when combined with regular exercise and spiritually uplifting therapies like yoga and t'ai chi—as outlined in *Mind Sense*—energy, vitality and real health will soon become the new norm.

Lack of exercise, pollution, hormones and stress don't help, which is where the supernutrients and superfoods come in. They help to mop up any toxin-induced damage, energize and keep body and mind strong, focused and completely in control.

A natural reaction to waning energy levels is to load the body with sugars and refined flour that give a rapid surge of energy. This is quickly followed by burnout, which over time leads to chronic fatigue, poor digestion and sleep disturbances. If, for example, you are suffering from lack of sleep, the first thing you will crave when you wake is a quick fix. However, if you persist with the preferred choices and opt for an extra protein meal, such as an egg white omelette (see page 50) or scrambled eggs, you will find your mind more focused and sharper throughout the morning. To prevent the afternoon slump or indeed tiredness at any time of the day, which is normally the result of

a drop in blood sugar levels, choose snacks like nuts, seeds or oatcakes. The protein content will revitalize both body and mind.

Gaining energy is not simply about physically fuelling the body. It also involves optimizing feel-good brain chemicals such as dopamine. This chemical helps keep the mind clear and positive. When dopamine levels slip, you are more likely to feel depressed, irritable and experience a loss of libido. Dopamine is made from the amino acid tyrosine—found in lean meat, pork, chicken, turkey, fish, eggs, pulses, almonds and peanuts—along with vitamin B12, also found in these foods. Folic acid, found in spinach, broccoli and other greens and fortified breakfast cereals, and magnesium in milk, nuts and seeds, also build dopamine. A diet packed with these brain-friendly foods ensures nourishing chemicals circulate continuously throughout the body.

Lack of iron is a common cause of low energy, especially in women. Eating more iron-rich foods such as lean meat, oily fish, peas, beans, lentils, spinach and other leafy greens and ready-to-eat dried apricots will help keep iron stores brimming with energy. Vitamin C helps the body make use of the iron from food, so ensure plenty of tomatoes, citrus fruits, kiwifruit and capsicums are part of your weekly plan. If you are chronically tired, a multivitamin and mineral supplement containing about 14 mg iron should be taken daily.

The beauty of time-honoured practices such as ayurveda and TCM is that they look beyond the physical to the emotional and physiological levels to find an explanation for imbalances in the system. This is especially relevant for the management of excessive anger and many stress-related conditions,

Rest and relaxation are important factors of any daily regime.
NEXT PAGE: Regular exercise, such as cycling or running, helps keep both your body and mind healthy, balanced and strong.

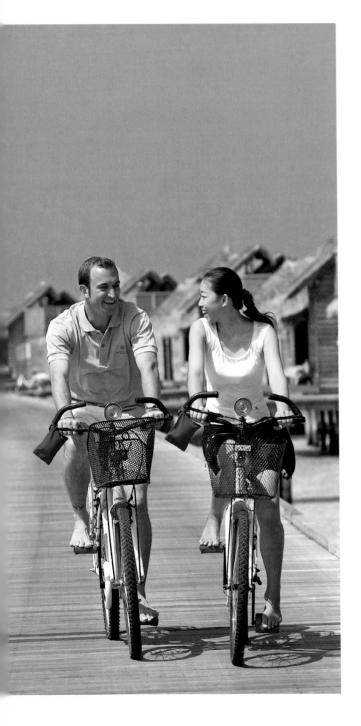

which are a leading cause of depleted energy and immunity. By living in harmony with nature's cycles and taking time to recognize what is happening from within, you can better maintain a more relaxed and open state and be more mentally empowered and spiritually alive. Along with yoga, t'ai chi, *qi gong* and pranayama, meditation will help you become more in tune with your inner thoughts and needs.

THE TRUE BENEFITS OF EXERCISE

Being fit does not necessarily mean being a top-level athlete. Real fitness is about being able to cope with the everyday physical demands of life while still having sufficient energy to deal with those occasional extra bursts. A healthy person should be able to run for a bus, dig strenuously in the garden or carry heavy bags without becoming too breathless. There are many reasons why regular exercise should make up a part of your *Balancing Senses* programme. Firstly, it helps you look better. Exercise increases blood flow to the skin, making you glow with health. Secondly, when combined with a healthy diet, it helps you to lose weight. The benefits are not always about how you look; exercise makes you feel happier. It releases endorphins or happy hormones, which will make you more relaxed and improve self-esteem. Exercising regularly will also give you a healthier heart by reducing the chance of high blood pressure, high cholesterol and obesity, all of which contribute to heart disease. Of course, exercise helps you become stronger by strengthening the bones and muscles and maintains joint mobility.

STARTING OUT

Weeks 1 and 2	Exercise
Monday	Walk/gentle jog. 30 minutes at a constant and steady pace
Tuesday	Yoga/t'ai chi. 45–60 minutes with 10 minutes pranayama or meditation
Wednesday	Pranayama
Thursday	Walk/gentle jog. 45 minutes at a constant and steady pace
Friday	Strength-building programme*
Saturday	Yoga/t'ai chi. 45–60 minutes with 10 minutes pranayama or meditation
Sunday	Rest

BUILDING PROGRAMME

Weeks 3 and 4	Exercise
Monday	Brisk walk/jog. 30 minutes followed by 15 minutes strength-building*
Tuesday	Yoga/t'ai chi. 45–60 minutes with 10 minutes pranayama or meditation
Wednesday	Pranayama
Thursday	Brisk walk/jog. 45 minutes at a constant and steady pace
Friday	Strength-building programme*
Saturday	Yoga/t'ai chi. 60–90 minutes
Sunday	Rest

* For an effective strength building programme, consult a personal trainer

Experts agree that the best way of approaching an exercise regime is integrating time-tested teachings from the East with more conventional sports science and medicine. Therefore a programme that combines spiritual therapies, such as yoga, t'ai chi and pranayama (see pages 121–7), that work both body and mind, with more Western-style cardiovascular activities that build strength, flexibility and endurance, will leave you physically and spiritually fitter and healthier. Try alternating 30 minutes gentle jog or brisk walk one day with an hour of yoga or t'ai chi the next. To many, exercise is a necessary evil on the road to long-term health, but it should be a positive experience. By combining different forms of exercise and activities, for example running, walking or swimming with yoga and t'ai chi, you are less likely to get bored and more likely to stick with your programme.

It is pertinent to remember that each of us is different, with our own unique requirements, so one regime won't work for everyone. If you are serious about achieving results, it is best to work with a reputable personal trainer and if you suffer from any medical or serious weight issues, consult your doctor before starting.

NATURAL IMMUNE BOOSTERS

Comprising the spleen, lymph nodes, thymus, tonsils, bone marrow and white blood cells, the job of the immune system is to fight off enemies—such as bacteria, viruses and cancer-causing free radicals—and repair any damage they cause. For boosting immunity naturally, think green. Packed with energy, vitality and antioxidants, greens are possibly the best investment for immune protection. In summer, choose salad greens, broccoli and spinach for

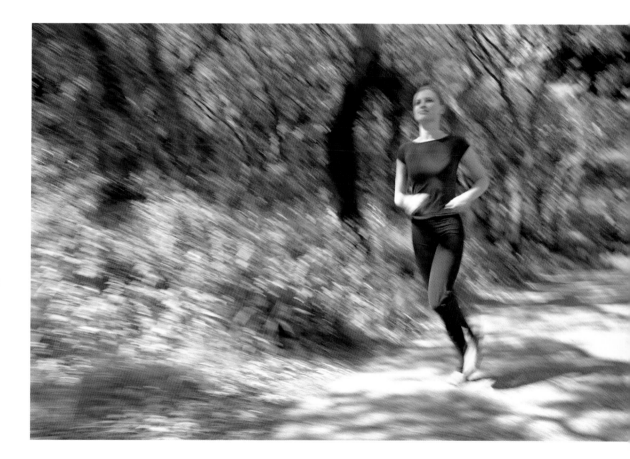

juices and meals. Cabbage, Brussels sprouts, bok choi and other Chinese greens are perfect winter boosters. Antioxidant-rich phytonutrients along with eggs, Brazil nuts, soya and turmeric help further scavenge free radicals and will help keep your immunity soaring.

Spirulina, a type of blue-green freshwater algae packed with vitamins and minerals, is a noted immune enhancer. Available from good health shops, it can be added to juices starting with 1 tsp per day, slowly increasing to 2–3 tsp.

Most of the juices outlined in the recipe section, featured later in this *Body Sense* chapter (see pages 72–3), contain natural

immune boosters but the Energizer, Memory Enhancer, Green Vitamin Booster and Summer Mint Magic will give an extra kick and can be added to any daily diet.

Effective stress management helps, too. Psychologists and self-help experts widely agree that what we believe, experience, think and feel has a powerful influence on the body's overall immunology. Hence a positive outlook on life keeps both body and mind strong and in complete control.

Other extras are probiotic supplements, antioxidant vitamins A, C, and E, zinc and selenium, as well as regular massage.

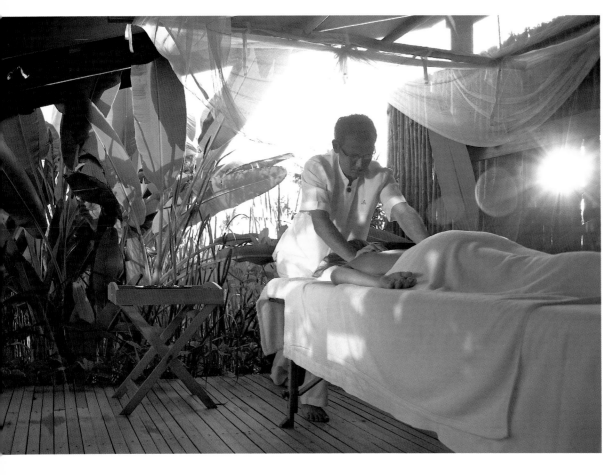

Massage relieves stress, tension and encourages sounder sleep.
OPPOSITE (FROM TOP): Deep sleep comes easily at Soneva Gili in the Maldives; 20 minutes of meditation every day is enough to keep you calm, relaxed and balanced.

BEATING STRESS Moderate stress is a positive reaction. In response to tricky situations and life's everyday stresses, the body releases hormones, such as cortisol and adrenaline, that sharpen the mind and give an extra burst of energy, allowing you to react rapidly and get through that crucial presentation, perform well or meet your deadline.

However, ongoing stress can trigger a number of problems from mood swings to depression, headaches, constant colds and infections. During stressful times, the nervous system needs extra supplies of B-vitamins to fight frustration, fatigue and the extra load placed on it. This is where food like porridge oats, barley and breakfast cereals fortified with minerals and vitamins, spinach, wheatgerm, apples and nuts become especially beneficial. Detoxing seasonally or after periods of overindulgence helps relieve built-up physical stress on the body as well as improving the way you feel about yourself. Otherwise, the *Balancing Senses* weekly plans (see pages 46–7) packed with stress-busting supernutrients combined with yoga, t'ai chi and meditation all contribute to unlocking stress, calming nerves and soothing pent-up tension.

A good night's sleep makes for a positively powerful day. Sleep is not an optional activity, but a biological imperative that does far more than simply rest the body. It heightens the senses, sharpens the mind and mellows the spirit. Lack of sleep leaves you feeling tired, on edge and more stressed. Although it is generally accepted that 8 hours sleep each night is the optimal amount, research has shown that the average person gets far less. When the body is in harmony, sleep will be deep and few dreams will be remembered.

'*If your stomach is uncomfortable, so will your sleep*' dictates the ancient Chinese scholars. In Chinese thinking, eating large meals late in the evening leads to stomach *qi* burnout resulting in heartburn, digestive problems and overall bed-time discomfort. The following are some simple measures for inducing sounder and deeper sleep patterns:

- Eat earlier and eat less, follow the 75 per cent rule (see page 19).
- Relax the heart first and then rest the eyes. Don't bring anger to bed.
- Exercise in the morning when the sun's yang energy is at its peak.
- Don't nap during the day.
- A warm milky drink or calming tea with lavender, camomile or peppermint help soothe both body and mind (see page 73).
- Keep the curtains open throughout the night to let the early morning sunlight fill the bedroom to stimulate wakefulness.
- Burn essential oils of lavender and camomile in the bedroom before going to bed.

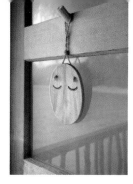

- A massage helps the body physically unwind.
- Aim to go to bed and rise at a similar time every day to keep your body balanced.
- A gently declining body temperature triggers the onset of sleep, so take a bath 1 hour or so before sleep.
- The bedroom should be as peaceful as possible and not too hot.
- Cut out stimulants such as caffeine, especially from the afternoon.
- Avoid strenuous exercise—other than sex— just before going to bed.

In Chinese medicine, daytime *qi* is active (yang), while at night *qi* is calm (yin). The body enters its yin phase after midnight when the yang *qi* takes time out to rejuvenate. Staying up past midnight works against these natural bio-circadian rhythms and is detrimental to our overall well-being. So, to keep in good health we should stay in tune with nature by sleeping during these calming night-time hours. Likewise, exercise is best performed early in the morning when yang is at its strongest and the body has more active energy.

CAFFEINE

Caffeine is a well-recognized nerve stimulant and if you are stressed it will further increase anxiety. Gradually cutting back, rather than cutting out all at once, will help to avoid painful withdrawal headaches and further stress. You will soon feel the benefits of calmer nerves.

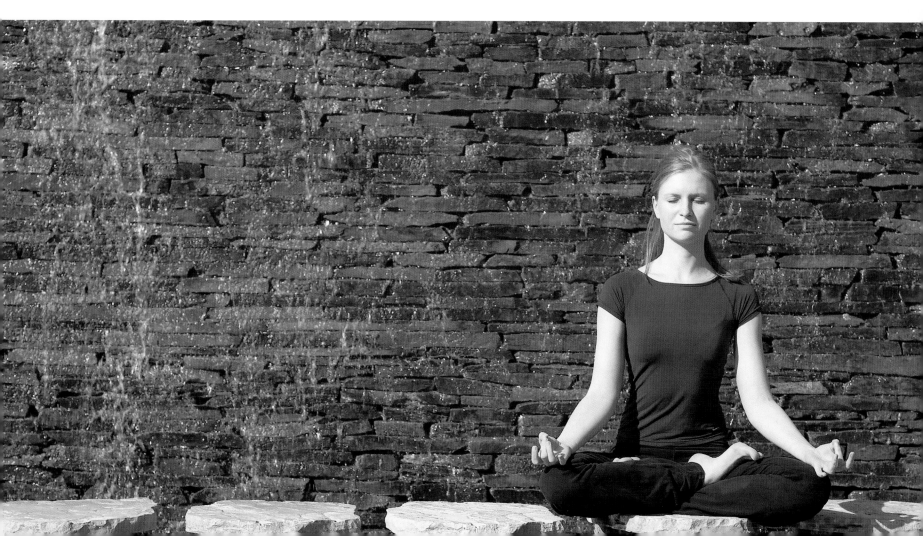

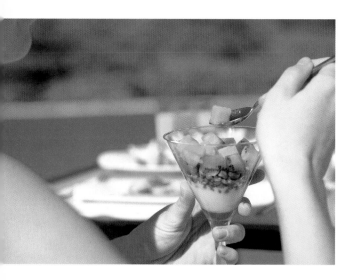

Fresh seasonal fruits served with nutrient-packed home-style muesli is the perfect start to the day.
OPPOSITE: Taking time for yourself will help you adjust to a new lifestyle.

THE GLYCAEMIC INDEX

The Glycaemic Index, or GI, is the healthiest and most successful route to long-term weight loss and overall health. Not that other diets don't work. Some do, but most come with built-in flaws which means that after a week or even a month, people simply cannot cope any longer and revert to their old eating habits that caused the problem in the first place. GI encourages you to eat well permanently.

The glycaemic index is a scale of 1–100 that measures the speed at which carbohydrates are digested in everything from bread, pasta and rice to cakes, sugar, cereals and fruit. When eaten, most carbohydrate must be digested and broken into its simplest form, glucose—with a GI score of 100—before passing through the walls of the intestine and into the blood to provide energy. Carbohydrates that are rapidly digested create a large increase in glucose levels in the blood and are said to have a high GI. Those that take longer to digest, releasing glucose more slowly into the blood, have a low GI. The backbone of GI eating is lots of low-GI carbohydrates.

The main problem with many foods today, especially with processed food, is while they may boast a reasonable nutrient and fibre intake they are bursting with sugar and fat. For example, many high-fibre breakfast cereals may indeed be low in fat, but are generally packed with sugar, sending blood sugar levels soaring. The sharp increase in the blood glucose level associated with eating high-GI, refined and processed foods, triggers the pancreas to release the hormone insulin, which instantly removes the excess glucose. This rapid removal has two effects. Firstly, the excess glucose ends up being stored in the muscles and liver and, once they are full, the excess is converted into fat and stored in the fat cells. Secondly, the consequent drop in blood glucose—or blood sugar—levels leaves the body feeling tired, hungry and craving more glucose. Conversely, eating low-GI foods causes a slower but steadier rise in the level of glucose in the body, which results in a smaller, more gentle rise in insulin. This keeps the body feeling satisfied for longer while also encouraging fat burn.

The closer the carbohydrate is to its natural state, the more likely it will have a lower GI. For example, unprocessed oats used in porridge and some muesli has a much lower GI than cereals where the grains are ground and processed. Also, breads with their fibrous outer husks intact, such as multigrain bread, are harder to digest than white bread, and will keep you feeling fuller for longer. In practical terms, it's simply a matter of replacing white rice with brown, wild or even black rice and white bread with multigrain and other less processed varieties.

High-GI foods have a GI score of 70 or more. These must therefore be avoided. Low-GI foods have a score of 55 and below, and medium-GI foods with a score of 56–69 can be eaten in moderation. Including low- and medium-GI foods in each meal will keep you feeling fuller for longer and will reduce the temptation to snack.

LIVING WITH THE GLYCAEMIC INDEX

- Switch to homemade breakfast cereals or those that contain bran or unprocessed oats or fruit-based breakfasts.
- Choose multigrain bread with seeds, barley and oats instead of plain white or brown.

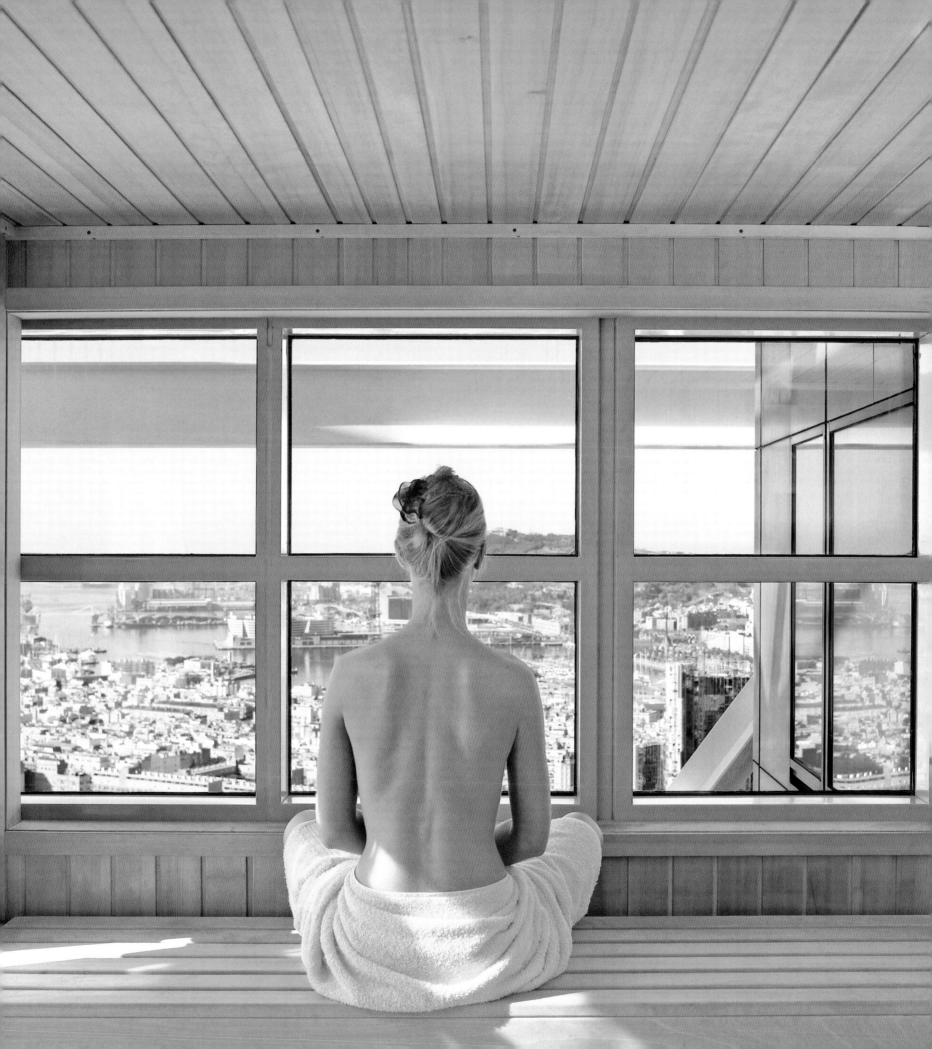

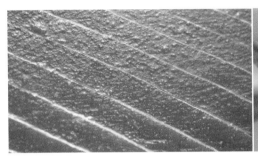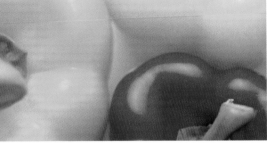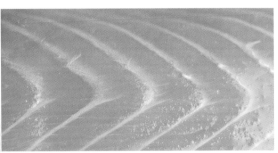

- Eat more wheat-based pasta and basmati rice instead of high-GI mashed potato and short-grain rice.
- Eat pulses and vegetables such as peas, lentils, chickpeas and soya products.
- Eat at least five portions of fruit and vegetables each day, choosing lower-GI options such as apples, dried apricots, grapefruit, grapes, oranges, peaches, pears and plums.
- Ensure the food you choose is more unrefined and unprocessed.
- Replace fruit juices with lower-GI fresh fruits or use the juice recipes outlined in the *Balancing Senses* recipe section (see pages 72–3).
- Include healthy protein-rich food such as lean meat, fish, tofu, beans, lentils, low-fat milk and dairy products with most meals.
- Cook vegetables lightly as overcooking increases the GI of the meal.

The acid in vinegar and lemon juice has been found to slow digestion by up to 30 per cent. Hence having a side salad with a tasty dressing reduces the overall GI of the meal. Also, the acid in sourdough bread, which is produced by the natural fermentation of starch and sugars by the yeast starter culture, has a similar effect, resulting in its low GI rating.

MAKING THE SWITCH

EAT MORE	EAT LESS
brown rice	instant rice
pasta/spaghetti	noodles
new potatoes	baked potatoes
sweet potato	mashed potato
oatmeal/oats/oatcakes	
pulses (beans, lentils)	tomato ketchup
plain nuts and seeds	
barley	
bulgur wheat	
porridge	cornflakes
bran cereal	rice cereal
green peas	
sweetcorn	
carrots	
green leafy vegetables	
grapes	watermelon
bananas	
under-ripe bananas	
oranges	
pears	
apples, apple juice	
grapefruit	
carrot and pineapple juices	
pumpernickel	baguettes
rye bread	bagels
sourdough bread	ciabatta
multigrain bread	white bread
	doughnuts
	biscuits
low-fat milk	
low-fat yoghurt	
peanuts/peanut butter	

Omega oil-rich tuna and salmon, and vitamin C-packed capsicums should be part of your diet.
OPPOSITE: Beef, nuts and eggs—all provide some of nature's nutrients.

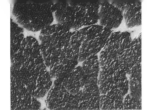

PROTEIN Protein is present in every cell in the body and accounts for about 16 per cent of our overall body weight. Protein helps speed up our metabolism—the rate at which the body burns calories—while in some ways it acts as a natural appetite suppressant, informing the brain that you have had enough and slows the digestion of carbohydrate foods. Protein-rich foods include meat, chicken, fish, eggs, dairy produce, soya, pulses and nuts.

FAT Although it's given very bad press, the good news fast gaining acceptance by many experts is that certain fats are in fact favourable. It is now accepted that some fats are packed with immune-boosting and anti-ageing goodness. What's more, they make food taste great and GI eating unquestionably encourages it.

BENEFICIAL FATS Fats from plants and fish are rich in essential fatty acids, or EFAs, which, just as the name suggests, are essential for health. Omega-3 and omega-6 are the good fats that form part of the wall of every cell in the body. One of the first places to show signs of EFA deficiency is the skin, which becomes flaky, dehydrated and wrinkled.

The typical human brain is 60 per cent fat and needs omega-3 for optimal function. In particular, omega-rich foods are believed to increase the number of connections between nerve endings or neurons and, in doing so, help the brain deal with thoughts and reactions more quickly and efficiently.

More recent research has implicated omega-3 in treating a range of psychiatric and neurological problems from schizophrenia to depression and Alzheimer's disease. While it is widely accepted that omega-3 fatty acids in

fish oils help prevent clots forming in the arteries, those who eat oily fish regularly have reduced risk of heart attacks and strokes. Recent studies suggest benefits beyond the heart. It's said fish oils aid the development of the nervous system and eyesight of a growing foetus during pregnancy and boost the level of concentration in growing children.

The richest sources of omega-3 EFAs are vegetable oils such as olive, hempseed and unrefined flaxseed oil, flaxseeds, fish—especially oily varieties like salmon, sardines, mackerel, fresh tuna and anchovies—leafy green vegetables and walnuts. Other foods, like eggs and dairy products, now come fortified with omega-3.

Omega-6 EFAs are found primarily in vegetable oils and just 2 tsp of sunflower, olive or corn oil or a handful of walnuts will give you your daily requirement.

HARMFUL FATS Both saturated and trans fats are detrimental to the body and not recommended in the GI or any other reputable healthy eating plan.

Most of the saturated fat eaten today is from animal sources such as fatty and processed meats—think sausages, burgers and meat pies, and full-fat dairy products such as

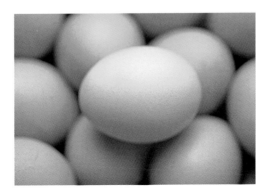

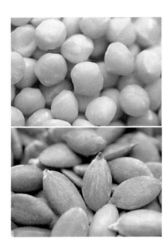

butter, cheese, cakes and pastries. Saturated fats have been shown to raise cholesterol levels in the body and increase the risk of heart disease and stroke.

Trans fat is a result of manufacturers adding hydrogen to vegetable oil. This hydrogenation process is used to increase the food's shelf life and flavour. Trans fats are also a result of the processing of plant oils into solid fats for the manufacture of cakes, biscuits, cereal bars and ready meals, among other foods. This artificial hardening of vegetable oils leaves some unhardened trans fats which cannot be digested by the body properly. Trans fat is now considered more harmful than the saturated fat it was designed to replace, and has been found to clog the arteries, thereby reducing the flow of blood and oxygen through the body. It can also block the links between the nerves in the brain, interfering with the way it sends messages.

When buying, always check the food label and avoid hydrogenated and saturated fats. Regardless of source, all fats are calorie dense—with 9 calories per gram—and should only be eaten in moderation.

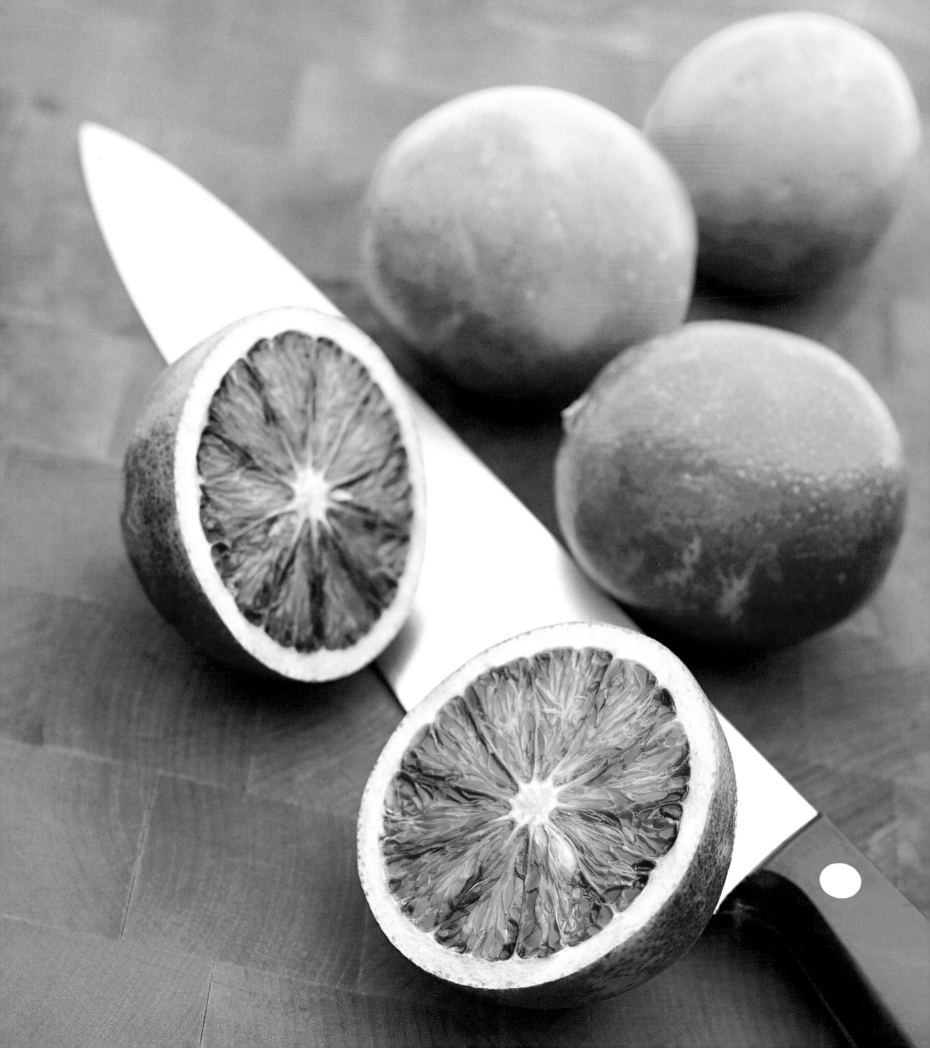

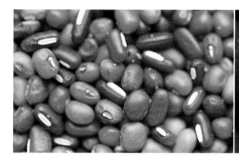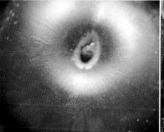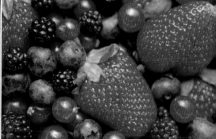

SUPERFOODS AND SUPERNUTRIENTS

Without doubt the best supplements for maintaining sleek, shiny hair, radiant skin and endless vitality are not pills, but superfoods that are naturally packed with powerful nutrients. Superfoods is the term used to describe these fruit, vegetables, nuts, seeds, fish and wholegrains that are alive with enzymes. These are whole foods that are powerhouses of vitamins, minerals, antioxidants—such as vitamins A, C, E, and trace elements of selenium and zinc. Also, phytonutrients, or plant chemicals, that are naturally present in fruit, vegetables, nuts and seeds have demonstrated favourable effects on health. These nutritionally high-powered foods are not new. What is new, however, is science's added knowledge about the disease-preventing components these nutrients contain. In today's polluted environment, these components are crucial protection that help to mop up free radicals, smoke and the general atmosphere. Further, these phytonutrients are said to offer the best natural protection against diseases such as cancer and heart disease.

Scientists have grouped phytonutrients into classes based on similar protective functions as well as individual physical and chemical characteristics. The most notable are as follows.

TERPENES AND CAROTENOIDS

Terpenes, found in green foods, soya and grains, comprise one of the largest classes of phytonutrients. Of these, carotenoids, which are the bright yellow, orange and red plant pigments found in vegetables like tomatoes, sweet potatoes, carrots, oranges, mangoes, pink grapefruit and spinach, are the most extensively studied. The yellow colour of egg yolk is due to carotenoids that protect the beneficial fat in the yolk. Over 600 naturally occurring carotenoids have been identified, and of these, beta-carotene—also known as pre-vitamin A—is the best known. Lycopene found in tomatoes is also a carotenoid. Their main role in the body is to protect skin cells from ultra-violet damage from the sun, to enhance the body's immune response and to help safely eliminate toxins.

PHENOLS

Phenols are found in blue-red and violet coloured foods—think berries, red grapes and eggplant—and protect plants and humans from oxidative damage. They help block specific enzymes that are responsible for inflammation and protect the heart by preventing blood platelets from clogging.

FLAVONOIDS

A sub-group of the phenol class with over 1,500 members, flavonoids are most commonly found in berry fruits, cranberries and grapefruit. Anthocyanidins, technically called flavonols, are a select group of flavonoids that provide links or bridges to connect and strengthen the strands of collagen protein through the body. Collagen is the most abundant protein making up soft tissues, tendons, ligaments, bone matrix and skin and its strength depends on the preservation of these cross-links. Anthocyanidins are also powerful scavengers of free radicals in tissue fluids and are

Red beans, plums and berry fruits are just some of the earth's natural superfoods that help improve health and well-being.
OPPOSITE: Oranges are packed with vitamin C and are the perfect partner to low GI eating.

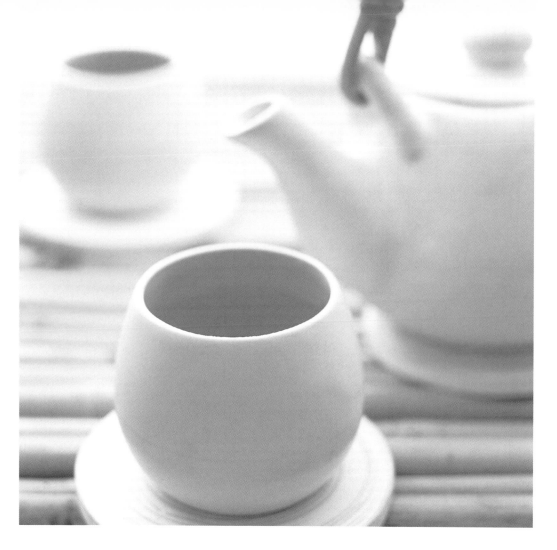

especially beneficial to athletes due to the amount of free radicals generated by exercise. Catechins, which are abundant in green tea, share the protective benefits of flavonoids.

ISOFLAVONES A sub-group of the phenol class and closely related to flavonoids, isoflavones are found primarily in soya products, beans and other legumes. They block the enzymes that are involved in the growth of tumours in the body. So effective is their protection, those who consume diets rich in soya products share a greatly reduced incidence of breast, uterine and prostate cancers.

ALLYLIC SULPHIDES Garlic and onions are the most potent members of this family, which also includes leeks, shallots and chives. Allylic sulphides come to life when the plants are cut or smashed, releasing their anti-carcinogenic, immune-boosting and cardiovascular benefits.

FERULIC ACID This potent antioxidant helps maximize the benefits of vitamins C and E, especially in skin protection from the sun and pollution. The key sources of ferulic acid are wholegrain cereals, berry fruits, apples, avocados, plums and corn-on-the-cob.

NATURE'S TOP SUPERFOODS

BLUEBERRIES When analysed for their antioxidant capabilities, blueberries gave the highest rating in their capacity to destroy free radicals. They are literally bursting with vitamin C, carotenoids and anthocyanidins that may help reduce the risk of cancer and lower the level of cholesterol. Besides this, their role in maintaining the strength of collagen protein makes blueberries the prefect prescription for glowing skin. If fresh blueberries are unavailable or price prohibitive, stock up on frozen as they have been found to retain 70 per cent of their vitamin C content as well as their protective antioxidants.

CRANBERRIES The antioxidants found in cranberries help flush the kidneys, thereby acting as a natural detoxifier.

FLAXSEEDS Naturally rich in omega-3 and omega-6 EFAs, as well as vitamin E, flaxseeds are a powerful antioxidant and help maintain healthy skin and hair while also supporting the immune system and protecting the body against the damaging effects of free radicals.

GREEN TEA Rich in antioxidant nutrients, green tea is the perfect partner during detox. Studies have shown that drinking five cups a day can burn off an extra 80 calories while the antioxidant catechins protect the skin from oxidative damage.

NUTS Dry roasted, unsalted or raw nuts, especially Brazil nuts, walnuts, almonds and pistachios, are rich in heart-healthy monounsaturated fats while also high in fibre, protein, vitamin E and phytochemicals.

OATS Brimming with heart-healthy goodness from antioxidants and fibre to vitamins and minerals, these low-GI power foods are currently the only wholegrain food recognized

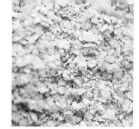

by the Food and Drugs Administration (FDA) in the United States to lower cholesterol and reduce the risk of heart disease.

CAPSICUMS These vegetables are an excellent source of vitamin C and carotenoids including beta-carotene that work to clear up free radicals from the sun and the environment.

PINEAPPLE Although rich in vitamin C and protective phytonutrients, it is the protein-digesting enzyme bromelain that makes pineapples especially useful for detoxing and gives them their superfood ranking.

POMEGRANATES Packed full with anthocyanidins that strengthen the skin's collagen and scavenge free radicals, pomegranates also keep the skin supple and prevent the formation of spider veins.

RED GRAPES The red pigment in grapes indicates an abundance of antioxidant anthocyanidins. Red grapes are also rich in ellagic acid, a natural antioxidant, and flavonols to cleanse the arteries.

GINGER High in magnesium, ginger acts as a natural hormone balancer for women. Drunk in tea, it is excellent for digestion while also calming the body and easing stomach upset (see recipe on page 73).

OILY FISH Salmon, tuna and other coldwater fish, for example mackerel and halibut, are packed with protein, vitamins A and D and minerals like selenium and zinc. However it's the high content of omega-3 EFA that gives these oily fish superfood status, and experts recommend that we eat at least two servings of these fish every week.

LEAFY GREENS Spinach and other leafy greens such as bok choi and broccoli are excellent sources of antioxidant vitamins C and E, beta-carotene, iron, calcium, potassium and B-vitamins, including folic acid. Calcium and potassium help maintain strong bones and contribute to healthy connective tissue. The B-vitamins help release energy from foods. Folic acid is an especially important member of the vitamin B family, most notably for women who are trying to conceive and during the first 3 months of pregnancy, as it helps prevent birth defects such as spina bifida.

TOMATOES The epitome of cancer-fighting superfoods, tomatoes are packed with vitamins A, C and E, fibre and lycopene, the antioxidant phytochemical—responsible for their rich red colour—which carry the dual benefits of protecting against cancer and heart disease.

WHEATGERM Nature's richest source of vitamin E also supplies magnesium, copper, calcium and phosphorus. Just a sprinkle of wheatgerm in cereals, yoghurts and cooking ensures you get your daily supply.

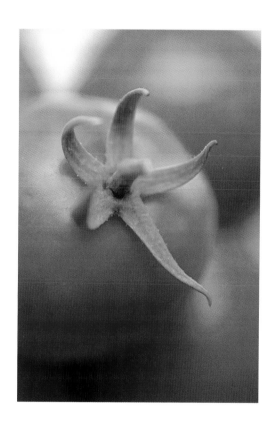

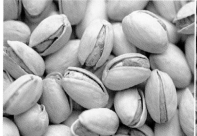
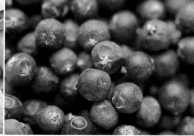
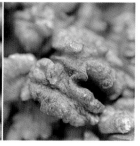

Wheatgerm, tomatoes, nuts and juniper berries, superfoods that boost health and vitality.
OPPOSITE: Green tea is an effective antioxidant that's popular the world over.

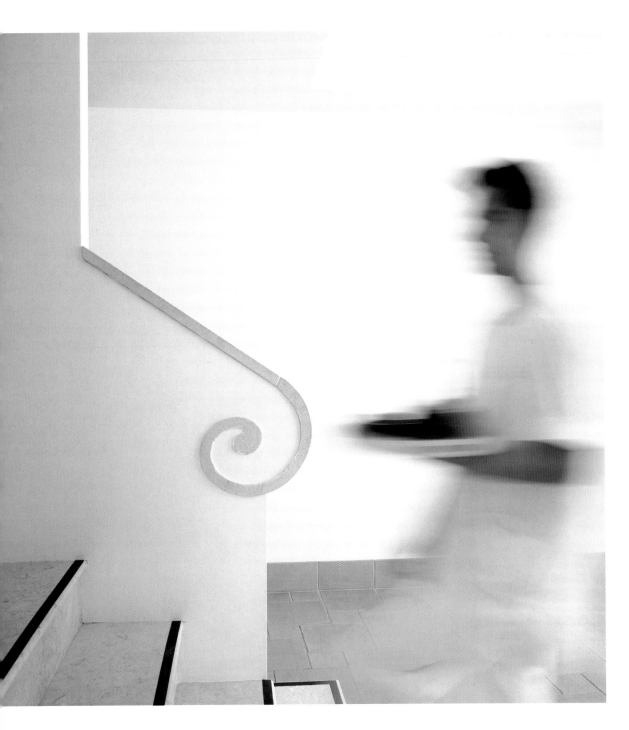

PROBIOTICS Irrespective of any extra efforts in hygiene, the average gut is oozing with 750 trillion bacteria and there's very little we can do about it. These essential, live bacteria, weighing about 1 kg / 2 lbs in the typical adult, make up the gut flora and are positively beneficial. They maintain a microbial balance by helping the immune system ward off more dangerous bacteria and assist in the breakdown of nutrients in the body.

As bacteria in the gut flora are constantly competing for nutrients and space, a normal healthy balance is easily upset, and problems such as diarrhoea, constipation and wind may result when harmful varieties take over. Overuse of antibiotics also destroys this internal synchronicity, as can skipping meals, stress and a super-refined diet that is low on fibre, fruit and vegetables and high in fast food.

Sadly, only a few types of probiotic bacteria are strong enough to resist attack by stomach acids and few survive the journey through the digestive system to reach the colon. Those that do include *lactobacilli* bacteria like *Lactobacillus acidophilus*, *Lactobacillus casei* and *bifido* bacteria like *Bifidobacterium bifidum*.

Probiotic-enriched foods and drinks such as live or bio-yoghurts rich in *lactobacilli* bacteria are now widely available and can help protect us; however some may not contain enough of the bacteria to lodge permanently in the body. When choosing a supplement, opt for one that provides at least 1 billion colony-forming units per serving. Yoghurt and fermented milks are other options that can be eaten or drunk daily in conjunction with a fibre-, fruit- and vegetable-rich diet as well as plenty of water.

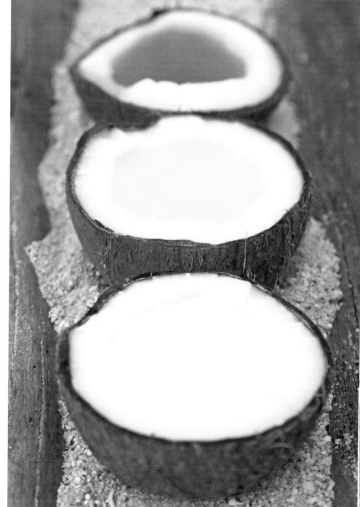

> Pumpkin, sesame and sunflower seeds ground in a blender in equal proportions makes a wonderfully versatile and vitamin packed complete protein to sprinkle on yoghurt, smoothies, salads and fruit.

BALANCING SENSES PYRAMID

A daily food intake should encompass the following food pyramid:

- 70 per cent fruit, vegetables and low-GI, unrefined carbohydrates.
- 20 per cent lean meat, chicken, oily fish, soya, eggs, pulses—such as peas, beans, and lentils—and low fat dairy produce.
- 10 per cent fats from fish and olive oil; there is also room here for some indulgent treats.

SIZE MATTERS Many studies have shown that the overall calorie intake of the average person is far too high, primarily because of larger portions. So, although it is not necessary to become preoccupied with counting calories at each meal, it is worth bearing an ideal portion size in mind. Think along the lines of an airplane meal.

For most people, calorie needs range between 1,500–2,000 per day. This need depends on the level of activity, age and body size and composition. By following the GI style of eating with emphasis placed more on complex carbohydrates, you will feel fuller for longer and weight loss or weight maintenance becomes much easier. However, eating too much of any type of food only makes matters worse. Variety is key. If weight loss is the ultimate goal, then regular exercise combined with a reduction in daily calorie intake is the answer to lifelong change.

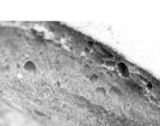

SERVING GUIDE

Each of the following is one serving:
BREAD 1 slice multigrain bread, 2 oatcakes, 1 pitta bread, 1 slice sourdough
POTATOES 180 g / 7 oz boiled new or baked sweet potato
PASTA AND RICE 70 g / 2½ oz uncooked pasta and 65 g / 2¼ oz uncooked brown or wild rice
FRUIT 1 medium sized fruit, such as an apple or pear, 3–4 dried apricots, 1 slice of pineapple, 3 prunes and 30 g / 1 oz sultanas and raisins
PROTEIN 40 g / 1½ oz cheese, 100 g / 3½ oz lean beef, pork or lamb, 80–100 g / 3–3½ oz oily fish, 150 g / 5½ oz tofu, 280 ml / ½ pint of low-fat or skimmed milk, 150 g / 5½ oz yoghurt, 100 g / 3½ oz cottage cheese
NUTS AND SEEDS 30 g / 1 oz

FROM LEFT: Yoghurt and fermented milks ensure that the body's gut flora remains balanced; The husk of a slice of multigrain bread keeps the GI score low. OPPOSITE: Therapists at the stylish Six Senses Spa at Penha Longa Hotel in Portugal assure complete rest and relaxation.

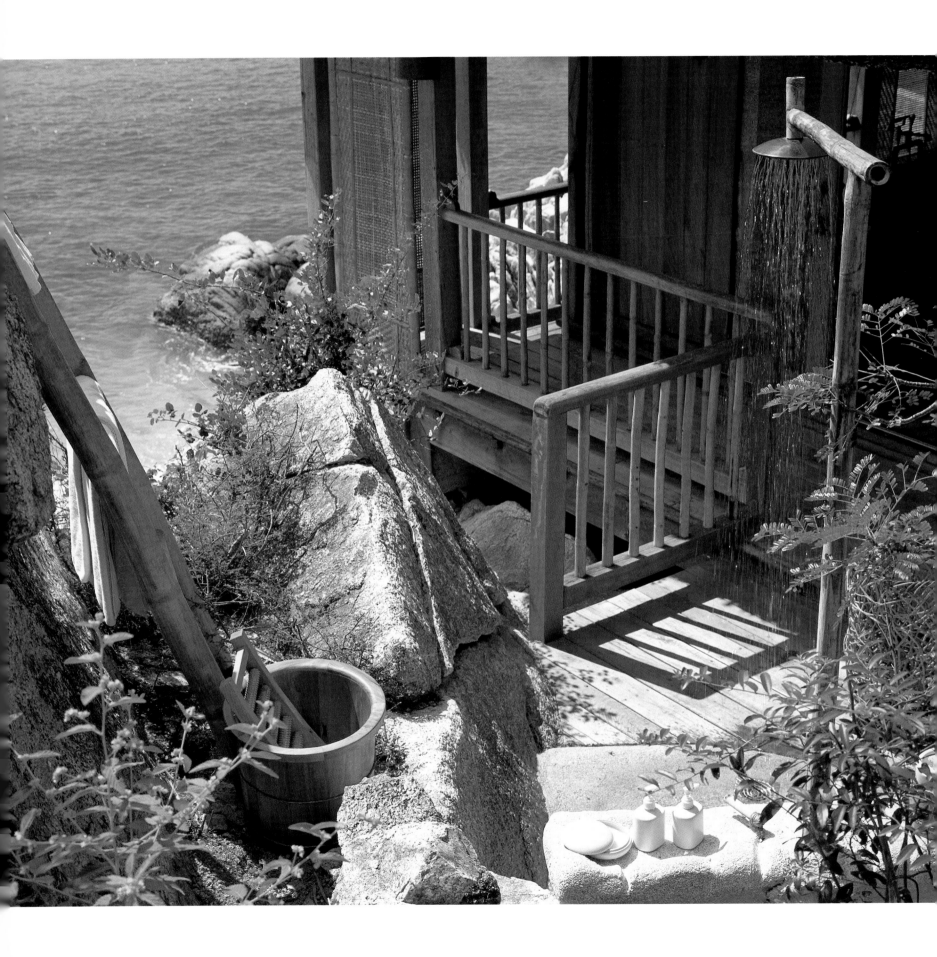

CLEANSING THE BODY Is your system overloaded? The body's primary elimination organs are the liver, kidneys, skin, bowel, lungs and lymphatic system. When they become overloaded they get sluggish and less efficient, with toxic symptoms starting to appear through the body. Detoxing is the body's spring-clean—it works by cleansing the organs, clearing toxic build-up and returning balance and harmony to the entire system.

SYMPTOMS OF IMBALANCE IN THE BODY

THE LIVER If there is an imbalance in the liver, you will suffer from bloating, nausea, indigestion and a furry tongue.

THE KIDNEYS If your kidneys are blocked or imbalanced, you will detect strong-smelling urine and a sluggish system.

THE SKIN AND FACE Congested, blotchy, dehydrated skin, dark circles under the eyes, bad breath and a furry tongue show an imbalance in the skin.

THE INTESTINE Abdominal problems such as constipation, gas and wind indicate imbalance in the bowel and intestine.

THE LUNGS A problem with the lungs will increase the likelihood of a runny nose, constant sneezing or sinus problems.

THE LYMPHATIC SYSTEM Frequent colds and flu, tiredness, cellulite and fluid retention will occur if the lymphatic system is run down.

Do not perform the following 10-day plan or liver flush if: you're unwell or recovering from illness; you're diabetic or have abnormal blood sugar levels; you are pregnant or breastfeeding; you are taking any medication or being treated by your doctor for any particular complaint.

SEASONAL DETOX

Chinese medicine maintains that eating with the seasons is crucial for ongoing health. For example, there is a certain time of the year when we should rest and recharge and a more appropriate time for detoxifying. In nature, the growth of plants reflects how the body's energy changes with the seasons. In Chinese thinking, energy rises and moves from within during the winter to the surface at spring, just as plants move from underground, tubers, upwards and out, above ground, spring greens. Greens are a traditional part of the spring diet in most cultures. Being plentiful and packed with chlorophyll, which absorbs energy from the sun, their use is associated with freshening, cleansing and rebuilding the body. So, spring is the ideal season for detoxifying a congested liver in preparation for the hot summer months (see Liver Flush on page 42).

Cherries, celery, beetroot, raspberries, strawberries, citrus fruits, apricots, cranberries, grapes, prunes and green tea are all excellent for stimulating the organs utilized during a detox session. The smoother the organs are working the better the metabolism and fat-burning abilities.

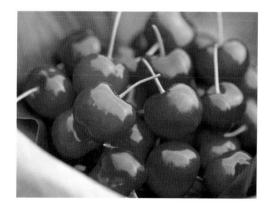

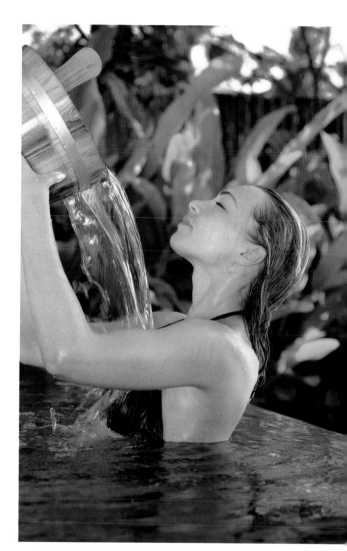

FROM TOP: Water is essential to life and bathing in cool, fresh water helps cleanse and purify the body; Fresh, cherries cleanse the organs from the inside during detox. OPPOSITE: The Hideaway at Ana Mandara offers great views as you shower in the garden of your Rock Villa.

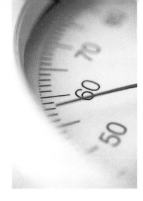

10-DAY CLEANSE

This is a time for you, so make the most of it. First really concentrate on calming the mind. Read, take baths, enjoy massage, yoga and t'ai chi, listen to calming music, burn soothing and cleansing essential aromatherapy oils such as lime, lemon and juniper. Even better, use some guided meditation CDs that will help start you on your journey to spiritual awareness through pranayama and meditation.

As with any successful detox, you may feel worse before you feel better, which is a sure sign that the body is cleansing. Keep with it, and focus on the body you want after the 10 days. The long-term results are well worth it.

BEFORE YOU START

Before starting any detox programme, stocking up on the daily essentials such as fruit, vegetables and herbs is essential. Try to buy as fresh and as colourful as possible to ensure meals are appetizing. Daily juicing is vital, so ensure you have a lot of detox juice ingredients on hand, along with a good juicer, some top quality extra virgin olive oil, plenty of fresh herbs, garlic and ginger.

Also, this is a good time to invest in some cleansing aromatherapy oils and a good quality body brush or loofah to brush and detoxify your skin with. The better you prepare, the easier your detoxing will be.

OTHER DAILY ESSENTIALS

- Probiotic supplement that provides at least 1 billion colony forming units per serving
- Multivitamin and mineral supplement
- Flaxseed oil, take 1 tsp per day
- Water, drink 1½–2 L / 1¾–2¾ pints of room-temperature-water

---

FOOD TO EAT DURING YOUR 10-DAY DETOX

Before you begin this 10-day detox programme, your newly stocked cupboards should contain a balanced mixture of low-GI items and superfoods and supernutrients (see pages 31–3). Together they will help your body to cleanse and make sure you feel completely renewed. Include the following ingredients on your shopping list.

FRUIT AND NUTS Apples, apricots, blueberries, cherries, kiwifruit, lemons, limes, papaya, peaches, pears, prunes, raspberries, strawberries, almonds and walnuts.

VEGETABLES Alfalfa sprouts, asparagus, beetroot, Brussels sprouts, capsicums, carrots, cauliflower, celery, chard, chives, eggplant, garlic, green beans, Jerusalem artichoke, leeks, onions, peas, pumpkin, spinach, cabbage and other members of the cabbage family, such as watercress, mustard leaves, horseradish, radish, kohlrabi, bok choi, choi sum and kale—spring onions, tomatoes, turnips and yams or sweet potatoes.

PROTEIN Skinless chicken and turkey, salmon and other oily and white fish such as tuna, and soya products such as miso.

GRAINS AND SEEDS Adzuki, or red beans, and other bean varieties, brown and wild rice, unprocessed oats, sunflower seeds and sesame seeds.

HERBS, SPICES AND CONDIMENTS Artichoke, basil, bay leaf, caraway, cardamom, cinnamon, chives, cumin, curry powder, dandelion greens, dill, fennel, ginger, honey, marjoram, nutmeg, olive oil, parsley, poppy seeds, rosemary, tarragon and turmeric.

DRINKS Green tea and herbal teas. (For the most ideal teas, see the detox recipes on page 73.)

While scales are a good indicator of weight loss, how you look and feel tells more about how healthy you are. OPPOSITE: Relaxing in water and soaking in the sun will do you a world of good, but always remember to protect your skin with sunscreen.

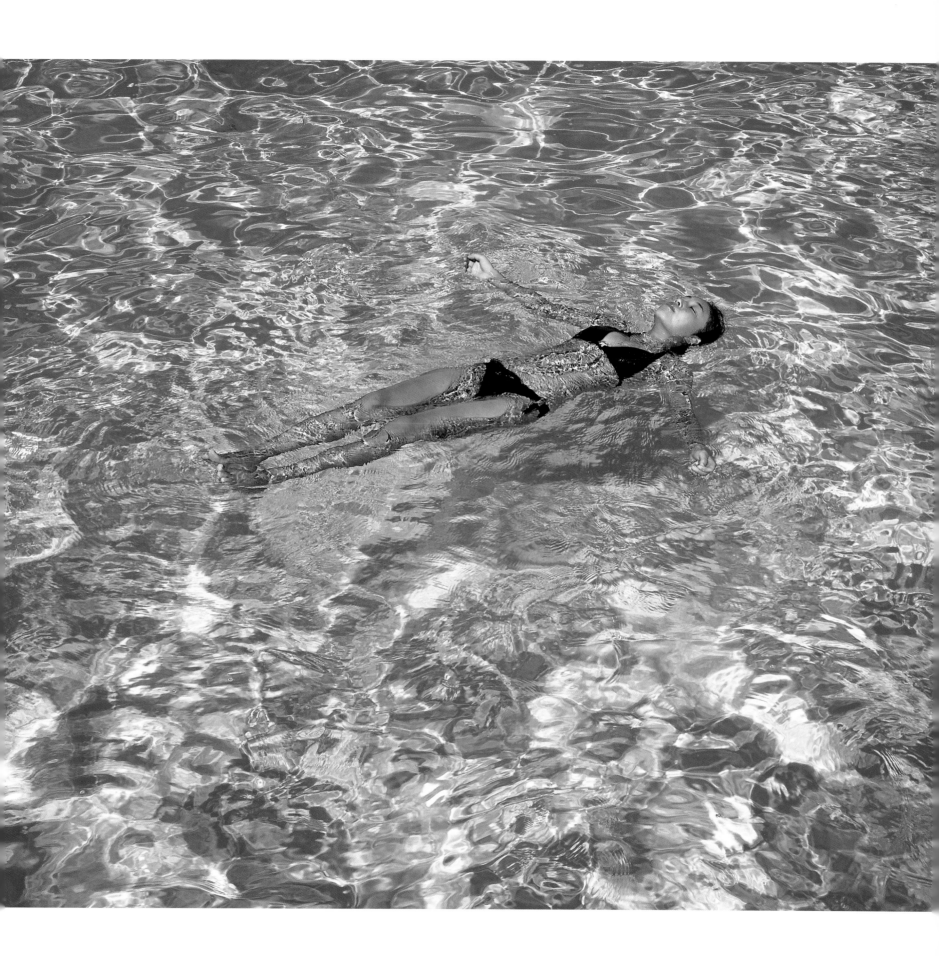

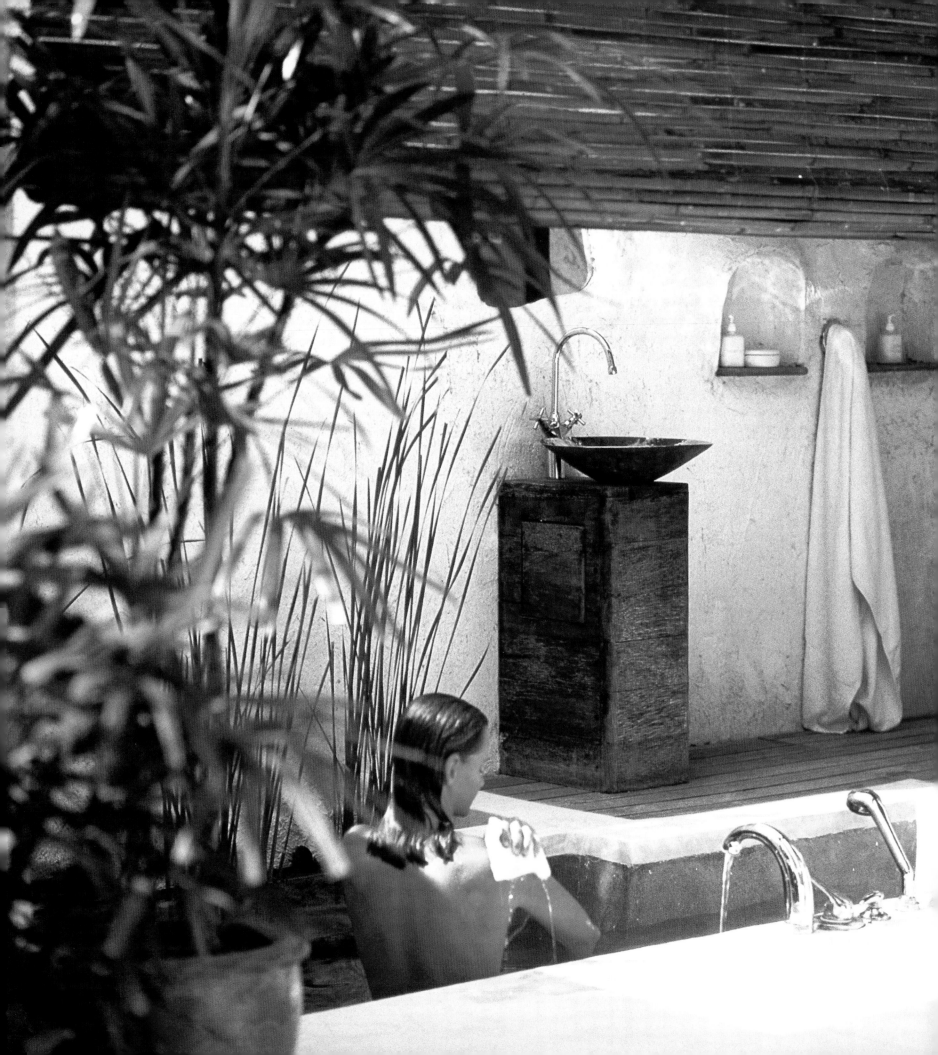

FOOD TO AVOID DURING DETOX

- Meat, milk and dairy products, excluding low-fat yoghurt
- Eggs
- Hydrogenated or trans fatty acids such as margarines, packaged and fast food
- Coffee, alcohol
- Peanuts and coconut products, although young coconut water is accepted
- Spicy foods, as they can upset the liver

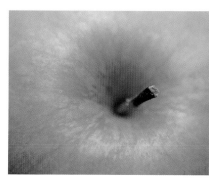
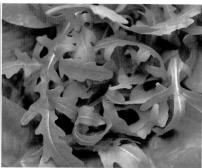
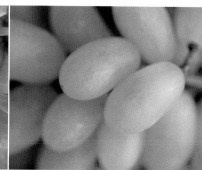

PLAN
All the following recipes are on pages 48–73

DAYS 1–3 THE UNLOADING PHASE

ON RISING
Drink a mug of warm water with lemon or lime juice. Honey can be added if desired.
Dry body brush before showering.

BREAKFAST
Blueberry Smoothie, Balanced Muesli or Bircher-Style Muesli with Berries (see page 48–9).
A large glass of juice from those suitable for detox (see page 72). This drink can be reserved until mid-morning if preferred.

MID-MORNING
1 serving of fruit and herbal tea

LUNCH
Detox Salad (see page 53)

MAIN MEAL
Chargrilled Tuna or Roasted Barracuda (see pages 58, 61) served with steamed green vegetables or tossed spinach leaves or Detox Salad; do not serve with rice.

DAYS 4–6 THE CLEANSING PHASE

ON RISING
Drink a mug of warm water with lemon or lime.
Drink another large glass of warm water with 1 tbsp Epsom salts.
Dry body brush before showering.

BREAKFAST
Large glass of Detox Juice or Salad in a Glass (see page 72)
Oat Breakfast (see page 49)

MID MORNING
1 kiwi fruit plus 1 pear or apple

LUNCH
Gazpacho or Mixed Vegetable Soup (see page 54)

MID-AFTERNOON
Large glass of V8, Salad in a Glass or tomato and wheatgrass juice

DINNER
On days 4 and 6: Delicious Detox Salad or large bowl of Gazpacho or Mixed Vegetable Soup.
On day 5: Steamed Salmon with Soya, Ginger and Chinese Black Mushrooms (see page 58) or Chargrilled Tuna served with steamed green vegetables or tossed spinach leaves; do not serve with rice.

DAY 7 THE LIVER FLUSH
(See page 42)

DAY 8–10 THE REBUILDING PHASE
Follow days 1–3 The Unloading Phase

Think green, apples, leafy greens and grapes will provide your body with supernutrients.
OPPOSITE: Before embarking on the detox plan, organize the days ahead and stock up on little luxuries, such as your favourite skin products, this will help the experience be more pleasurable.

DETOX, AYURVEDIC STYLE

Not for the faint-hearted, panchakarma is one of ayurveda's most effective regimes for full detoxification therapy. Comprising several steps, panchakarma involves the complete removal of toxins at the deepest internal levels with the aim of rebalancing the body's inherent equilibrium and doshas. This treatment can be prescribed either as individual treatments or as a combination depending on individual requirements. Therapy normally takes a minimum of two weeks and is not advised for those suffering from anaemia or weakness, pregnant women, or the very young and elderly.

Purvakarma is the pre-operative phase of panchakarma, comprising oil and sweat therapy to soften and cleanse the skin in preparation for detoxification. The five phases of detoxification are vamana or emetic vomiting induced through consumption of special potions; virechana or gentle purging with herbal tea; vasti or enema: nasya or nasal scenting where a few drops of medicated oil are applied to the nose to clear the nasal passages and alleviate imbalances such as headaches, allergies, sinusitis and nasal congestion; and raktamokshana or blood-letting where surgical instruments or leeches are used to drain the body of impure blood.

Panchakarma really works, but should only be followed under very close medical supervision. It is generally administered in destination retreats which specialize in ayurvedic medicine.

Just 5 minutes of body brushing a day helps breakdown congestion and stimulate the body. OPPOSITE: The ingredients for a successful liver flush that will leave your body renewed and energized.

THE LIVER FLUSH

Flushing the liver is believed to improve digestion, help eliminate allergies, and ease shoulder, abdominal and upper back pain. Furthermore, you will see increased energy levels and a sense of overall well-being. Following this programme will clear stagnation in the liver and is ideally carried out at the end of the first week of cleansing. It can also be repeated to coincide with seasonal change, after periods of excess or to further weight loss, but should not be carried out more than four times per year. Liver flushing is best done over a weekend or when you have a complete rest day as you will need to stay close to a bathroom. After the two-day programme, don't be surprised if you pass small stones that may have formed in the liver.

YOU WILL NEED

1 bottle virgin olive oil
6 lemons
60 g / 2¼ oz Epsom salts
3 L / 5¼ pints of water

DAY 1

To prepare for the Liver Flush, drink fruit juices for breakfast and juice or soup for lunch on the first day. Be sure to drink at least 1½ L / 2¾ pints of water during the afternoon before doing the following:
6.30 pm: Drink 1 heaped tbsp Epsom salts mixed into a large glass of warm water.
7.30 pm: Repeat 6.30 pm stage, followed by a few mouthfuls of water to rinse. Shower and dry, then body brush in an upward motion towards the heart.
8.30 pm: Squeeze 6 lemons to get approximately 100 ml / 3½ fl oz pure lemon juice. Add this to 200 ml / 7 fl oz olive oil, at room temperature, and blend together. Over

the following 1½ hours drink this mixture, about a quarter at a time, until finished. When in bed, lie on the left side to keep the liver clear.

DAY 2

6.30 am: Drink 1 heaped tbsp Epsom salts mixed into a large glass of warm water. You can start to eat light food after 8.00 am, but do not stray far from the bathroom.

DETOXING EXTRAS

BODY BRUSHING This gentle yet powerful technique breaks down congestion by stimulating internal movement and draining the lymphatic system. Just 5 minutes in the morning before showering, always brushing towards the heart, makes a big difference.
SAUNAS Dry saunas promote sweating and the release of fat-soluble toxins through the skin. It is recommended to stay in the sauna for a minimum of 30 minutes, inclusive of short breaks, so the temperature must not be excessive. Shower well afterwards to ensure toxins are completely removed. Take flaxseed oil daily to replace lost essential fats.

Don't expect to look completely different after just 10 days—but you will feel lighter, brighter, energized and more alive.

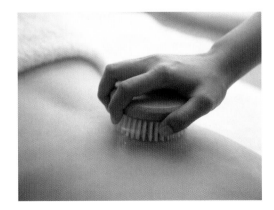

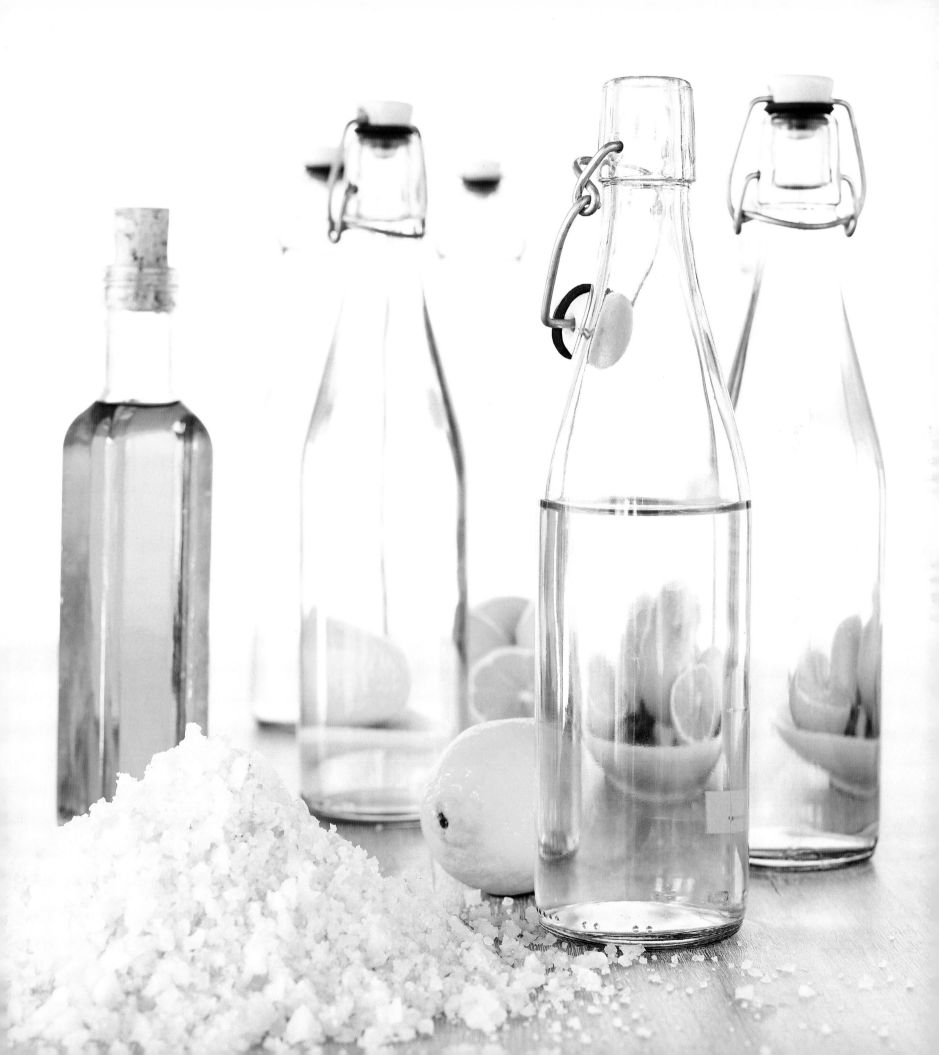

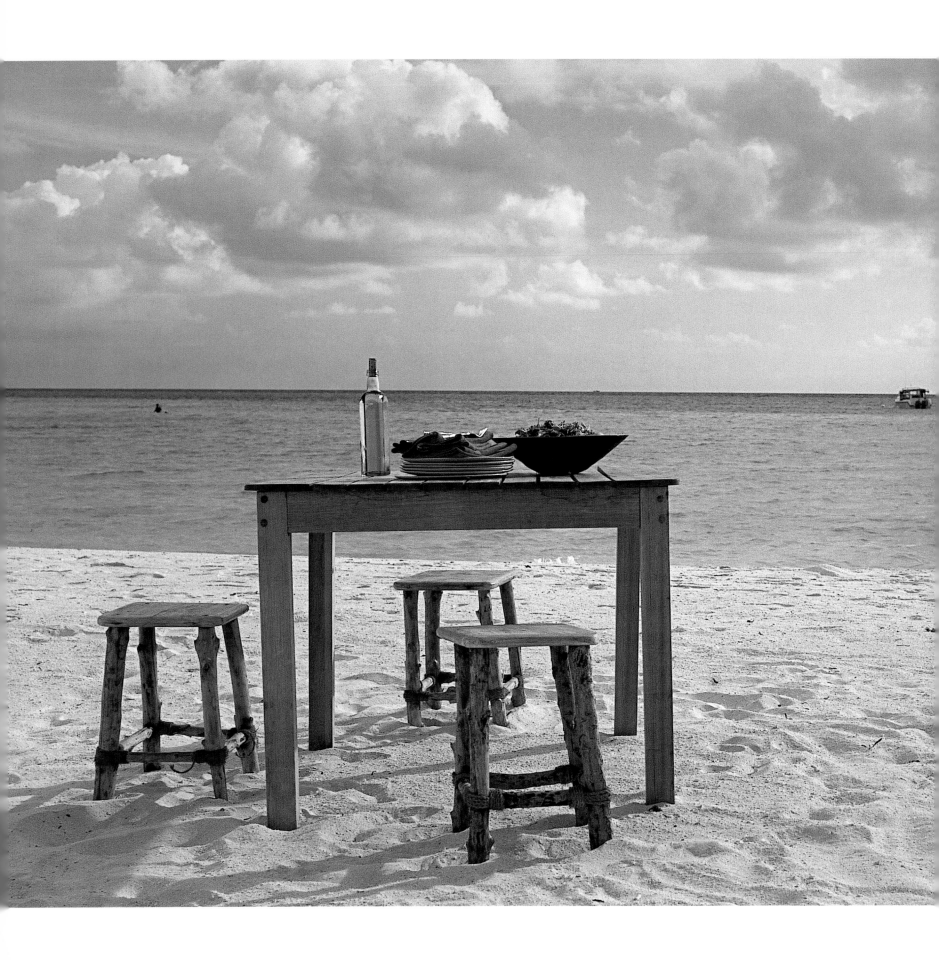

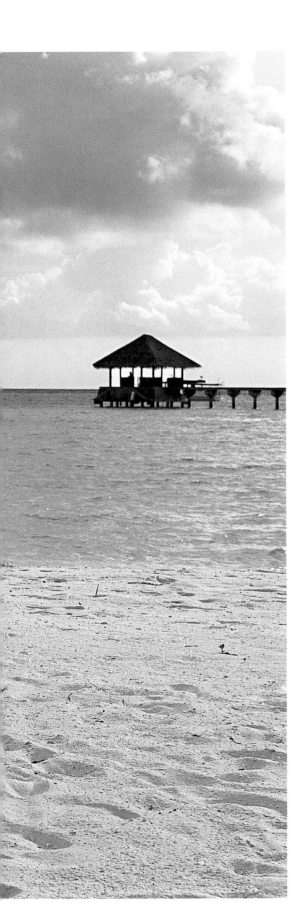

BALANCING SENSES FOR LIFE

Now that you are cleansed and energized, use your knowledge of supernutrients, GI and fresh, seasonal foods to get you on your way to lifelong health with the following weekly plans. Don't be too rigid; it is to help you on your way. If you do not eat or enjoy meat for instance, simply replace that recipe with another main course more to your liking. It is worth preparing the salt substitute and other herb and spice mixes; they can be stored and are on hand when called for in recipes. Always have plenty of fruit, vegetables and herbs on hand. Even better, grow your own herbs. You don't need to have a garden; a window box is perfect.

EATING OUT This is a pleasure we should all enjoy. If it is a regular part your lifestyle, it is no excuse not to eat well. Rather the reverse, as you don't have to prepare the food and can sit back and make the most of it. You can still eat *Balancing Senses*-style by just keeping the supernutrient and low GI secrets in mind.

Try not to arrive at the restaurant feeling ravenous; have a small snack before you leave. If the breadbasket tempts you, ask for some olives to pick at before your meal.

When choosing meals, go back to basics with a salad, homemade soup or plain fish as a starter. Follow this with grilled or roast lean meat, chicken or game, or grilled or baked fish with lots of fresh vegetables or salad as a main. Always ask for the dressing or sauce on the side. For an added kick, spice-up a dish with mustard or chilli sauce. Don't be afraid to make special requests. Most restaurants are happy to oblige. To end a meal, choose a fruit-based dessert or a herbal tea with a small piece of chocolate. Above all, enjoy.

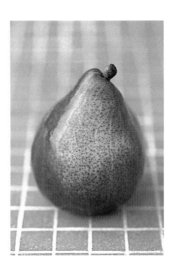

Pears are packed with roughage and vitamins and make an ideal *Balancing Senses* snack food.
OPPOSITE: Dinner on the beach, the perfect end to the perfect day at Soneva Gili in the Maldives.

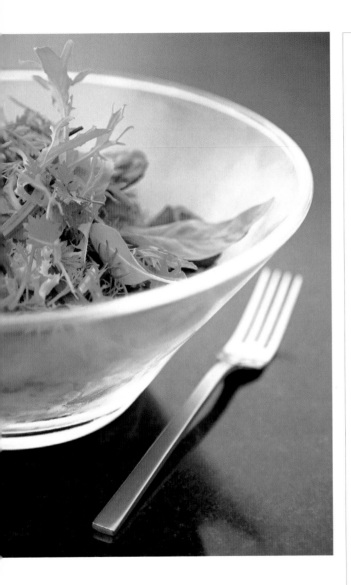

WEEK 1: MONDAY

BREAKFAST
Energetic Morning

LUNCH
Chilled Rice Salad

MAIN MEAL
Grilled Chicken with Tomato-Avocado Salsa
and lightly steamed vegetables or salad

WEEK 1: TUESDAY

BREAKFAST
A detox juice with Egg White Omelette

LUNCH
Pitta pocket packed with salad greens and a
serving of feta or goat's cheese

MAIN MEAL
Chermoulah Spiced Sea Bass or Roasted
Barracuda with organic tossed spinach leaves

WEEK 1: WEDNESDAY

BREAKFAST
Energizer Juice with Balanced Muesli

LUNCH
Zucchini, Rocket and Scallop Salad or
Simple Healthy Spinach Salad

MAIN MEAL
Mediterranean Pasta, followed by dessert
of your choice

WEEK 1: THURSDAY

BREAKFAST
Juice of your choice with Fruit Bran Milk Shake

LUNCH
Soup of your choice with multigrain sandwich
packed with Sandwich Filler

MAIN MEAL
Wok-Fried Chicken with Ginger and Sesame
served with wild rice

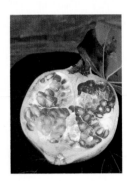

WEEK 1: FRIDAY

BREAKFAST
A detox juice with Bircher Muesli with Berries

LUNCH
Tian of Avocado and Wild Rice

MAIN MEAL
Steamed Salmon with Soya, Ginger and
Chinese Black Mushrooms, followed by dessert
of your choice

WEEK 1: SATURDAY

BREAKFAST
Blueberry Smoothie with
Wholewheat Pancakes

LUNCH
Tartare of Wild Salmon with
Spiced Yoghurt Relish

MAIN MEAL
Crunchy White Snapper with a Pistachio,
Macadamia & Coconut Crust

WEEK 1: SUNDAY

BRUNCH
Juice or Smoothie of your choice followed by
two poached or scrambled eggs on a slice of
toasted multigrain or warm sourdough bread

MAIN MEAL
Lamb Osso Bucco with Thai herbs served with
rice and sautéed spinach, followed by dessert
of your choice

ALCOHOL

For those who enjoy it, there is no reason why
alcohol should not be included in eating the
Balancing Senses way. It is good for you, in
moderation. However, it does contain calories
so, if you are trying to lose weight, it is best
avoided with maybe the very occasional glass of
wine. From a health perspective, the good news
is that alcohol in moderation has been found to
protect the heart and, as an added bonus, it
de-stresses the mind after a chaotic day.

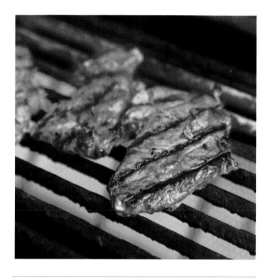

WEEK 2: MONDAY

BREAKFAST
A juice with Oat Breakfast

LUNCH
Pitta pocket packed with salad greens and a serving of feta or Goat's Cheese with Tomato Conserve, Tomato and Rocket Jus

MAIN MEAL
Chargrilled Tuna with lightly steamed vegetables or a large salad

---

WEEK 2: TUESDAY

BREAKFAST
A detox juice with Egg White Omelette

LUNCH
Seafood and Tropical Fruit Ceviche or Goat's Cheese with Tomato Conserve, Tomato and Rocket Jus

MAIN MEAL
Mediterranean Pasta, followed by dessert of your choice

WEEK 2: WEDNESDAY

BREAKFAST
Energizer Juice with Balanced Muesli

LUNCH
Simple Healthy Spinach Salad

MAIN MEAL
Wok-Fried Chicken with Ginger and Sesame with wild rice

WEEK 2: THURSDAY

BREAKFAST
A juice with Fruit Bran Milk Shake

LUNCH
Open sourdough sandwich with Sandwich Filler or feta cheese and salad greens

MAIN MEAL
Lamb Osso Bucco with Thai Herbs served with rice and sautéed spinach

WEEK 2: FRIDAY

BREAKFAST
A detox juice with Bircher Muesli or Oat Breakfast with mixed berries

LUNCH
Tian of Avocado and Wild Rice or Chilled Rice Salad

MAIN MEAL
Steamed Salmon with Soya, Ginger and Chinese Black Mushrooms, followed by dessert of your choice

---

WEEK 2: SATURDAY

BREAKFAST
A juice with Blueberry Smoothie or Wholewheat Pancakes

LUNCH
Large bowl of Gazpacho Soup with a slice of warm sourdough bread

MAIN MEAL
Mediterranean, or other vegetarian, Pasta

WEEK 2: SUNDAY

BREAKFAST
Poached Fruit followed by a boiled or poached egg and a slice of multigrain or sourdough bread

LUNCH
Tartare of Wild Salmon with Spiced Yoghurt Relish or Seafood and Tropical Fruit Ceviche

MAIN MEAL
Roast Beef with baked baby potatoes and marinated vegetables, followed by dessert of your choice

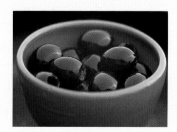

SNACKS

A handful of mixed plain nuts and seeds
- 200 g / 7 oz low-fat plain or fruit yoghurt
- All fruit except watermelon
- Vegetable crudités with hummus
- A handful of olives with a small chunk, or matchbox-sized piece, of feta
- A slice of sourdough or rye bread topped with either a slice of cheese or 2 tsp of crunchy peanut butter*
- A slice of pumpernickel bread topped with a thin spread of low-fat cream cheese or a slice of hard cheese
- A handful of dried apricots
- A juice or smoothie from recipes
- A small bowl of soup from recipes
- A serving of poached fruit
- A small homemade wholewheat muffin*
- A small portion, 20 g / ¾ oz, of chocolate, preferably dark, as an occasional treat*

* these are higher in calories; take in moderation when trying to lose weight

Chicken is a great source of protein; A handful of olives makes a healthy snack.
OPPOSITE: Salad with dressing will get the appetite going; Pomegranates are superb detoxifiers that mop up pesky free radicals.

ENERGETIC MORNING Serves 2

250 ml / 9 fl oz / 1⅛ cup low-fat milk
4 tbsp low-fat yoghurt
Juice from 2 punnets of strawberries
2 passionfruit
2 tsp wheatgerm
2 tsp wild honey

Combine all ingredients in a blender until smooth
and serve immediately.

BLUEBERRY SMOOTHIE Serves 2

3 handfuls of blueberries
250 ml / 9 fl oz / 1⅛ cup fresh unsweetened
pineapple or orange juice
250 g / 9 oz low-fat yoghurt
1 tsp wild honey

Combine all ingredients in a blender until smooth
and serve immediately.

FRUIT BRAN MILK SHAKE
Serves 2

600 ml / 1 pint / 2½ cups skimmed milk
200 g / 7 oz All Bran cereal
½ tsp ground cinnamon
Seeds of 2 vanilla pods
2 green apples, sliced

Freeze three quarters of the milk in a cube tray
overnight. Place the All Bran, cinnamon, vanilla pod
seeds, and apple into a blender. Add the remaining
milk and blend for 20 seconds. Continue blending
while slowly adding the frozen milk cubes (you
may not need all). Taste and adjust accordingly
before serving.

Energetic morning;
Blueberry smoothie; Fruit
bran milk shake.
OPPOSITE (FROM LEFT): Balanced
muesli; Bircher-style muesli
with berries; Oat breakfast.

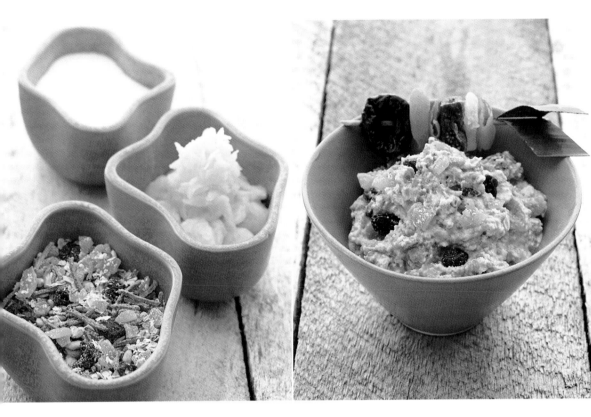
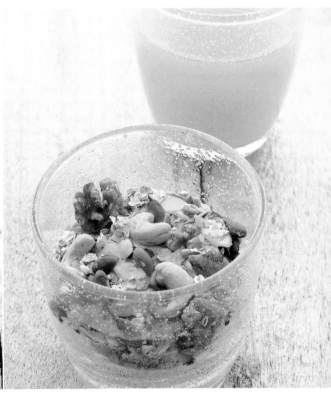

BALANCED MUESLI Serves 2

60 g / 2¼ oz bran flakes
2 tbsp chopped dried apricots
2 tbsp rolled oats
2 tbsp sunflower seeds
1 tbsp wheat bran
1 tbsp seedless raisins
1 tbsp wheatgerm
1 green apple, cored and grated
or 1 banana, sliced
250 g / 9 oz low-fat yoghurt

Combine bran flakes, dried apricots, rolled oats, sunflower seeds, bran, raisins and wheatgerm. Store in an airtight container in the refrigerator. To serve, top with grated apple or sliced banana and yoghurt to moisten.

BIRCHER-STYLE MUESLI WITH BERRIES Serves 2

4 tbsp soya milk
30 g / 1 oz rolled oat flakes
2 tsp oatmeal
120 g / 4¼ oz plain fromage frais
2 tsp wild honey
2 small green apples, grated
10–12 walnuts, chopped
200 g / 7 oz mixed berries, raspberries, blueberries, strawberries
2 tsp sunflower seeds

Warm soya milk and pour over combined oats and oatmeal. Leave to soak overnight in the refrigerator. To serve, stir in fromage frais and honey. Combine apple with walnuts and berries and add to oat mixture. Sprinkle over sunflower seeds and serve.

OAT BREAKFAST Serves 2

60–80 g / 2¼–2¾ oz rolled oats
4 tbsp unprocessed roasted nuts (almonds or walnuts), chopped
60 ml / 2 fl oz guava juice mixed with 40 ml / 1½ fl oz water (use fresh unsweetened pineapple, papaya or apple juice if guava juice is unavailable)
2 tbsp wild honey (omit during detox)

Place oats and nuts in a bowl. Stir in guava juice-water mixture and mix well. Add as much liquid as required to make a porridge consistency. Add honey if desired, but not during detox.

EGG WHITE OMELETTE Serves 2

10 egg whites
2 whole eggs
40 g / 1½ oz bean sprouts
1 bird's eye chilli, seeds removed, chopped
Small bunch of coriander leaves, chopped
2 spring onions, chopped
Herbal salt substitute (see recipe on page 75), to taste
Freshly ground black pepper, to taste

Mix egg whites with 2 whole eggs and fold raw vegetables into the mixture. Pour into a shallow pan, over a medium heat using as little oil as possible, and cook briefly maintaining the freshness of the vegetables. Serve immediately. For lunch, a side salad of mixed greens with herbs (without dressing) makes a complete meal.

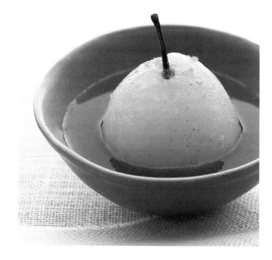

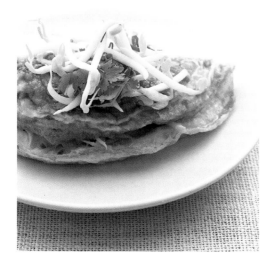

POACHED FRUIT Serves 2

2 pears, apples or peaches (1 piece per serving)
Juice of 2 limes or lemons in 800 ml / 1⅓ pint cold water
1 L / 1¾ pint / 4 cups water
Peel of 2 oranges
Peel of 1 lime
1 vanilla pod
4 tbsp wild honey

Peel pears, apples or peaches and place in cold water with lime or lemon juice to stop fruit from browning. In a saucepan place the other 1 L / 1¾ pint / 4 cups of water, orange and lime peel, vanilla pod, and honey and bring to a boil. Add the peeled whole fruit to the pan, reduce the heat to low and cook for 25 minutes. Remove pan from heat and allow to cool. To reduce calories, honey can be omitted. The poached juice can be kept in the refrigerator for up to 5 days.
A quicker alternative is to cut fruit into bite-size chunks. Prepare juice as above, with either 2 slices of ginger or 2 sliced lime leaves per piece of fruit, or 1 stalk of lemongrass chopped with a little honey. Add chopped fruit to the juice, cover and simmer on a low heat, frequently tossing the pan, for about 5 minutes. Remove pan from the heat and allow to cool. Store in the refrigerator until ready to serve.

WHOLEWHEAT PANCAKES
Serves 2

2 tbsp wild honey
80 g / 2¾ oz wheatgerm
160 g / 5½ oz wholewheat flour
2½ tsp baking powder
350 ml / 12 fl oz / 1½ cups low-fat milk (or soy milk)
2 tbsp vegetable oil
100 g / 3½ oz low-fat cottage cheese

In a large non-stick frying pan, heat honey over a medium–low heat until it becomes watery. Add wheatgerm and stir. Raise heat to medium–high to toast wheatgerm to a golden brown colour with a nutty aroma. Set aside to cool. In a large bowl, sift wholewheat flour and baking powder together. Add flour to wheatgerm and honey mixture and stir thoroughly. In a separate bowl, combine milk and oil. Add wet ingredients to dry and stir until the two are well mixed. Add cottage cheese to make the mixture slightly lumpy. Over a medium heat, add 2 tbsp of the pancake mixture into the frying pan and cook for about 2–3 minutes, or until small bubbles appear. Flip and cook the other side for another 2 minutes, or until pancake is golden brown. Pancakes can be served with a filling of nuts, sliced apple or pear and raisins. The batter can also be seasoned with vanilla, cinnamon or cardamom for added flavour.

Egg white omelette;
Poached fruit.
OPPOSITE: Wholewheat pancakes.

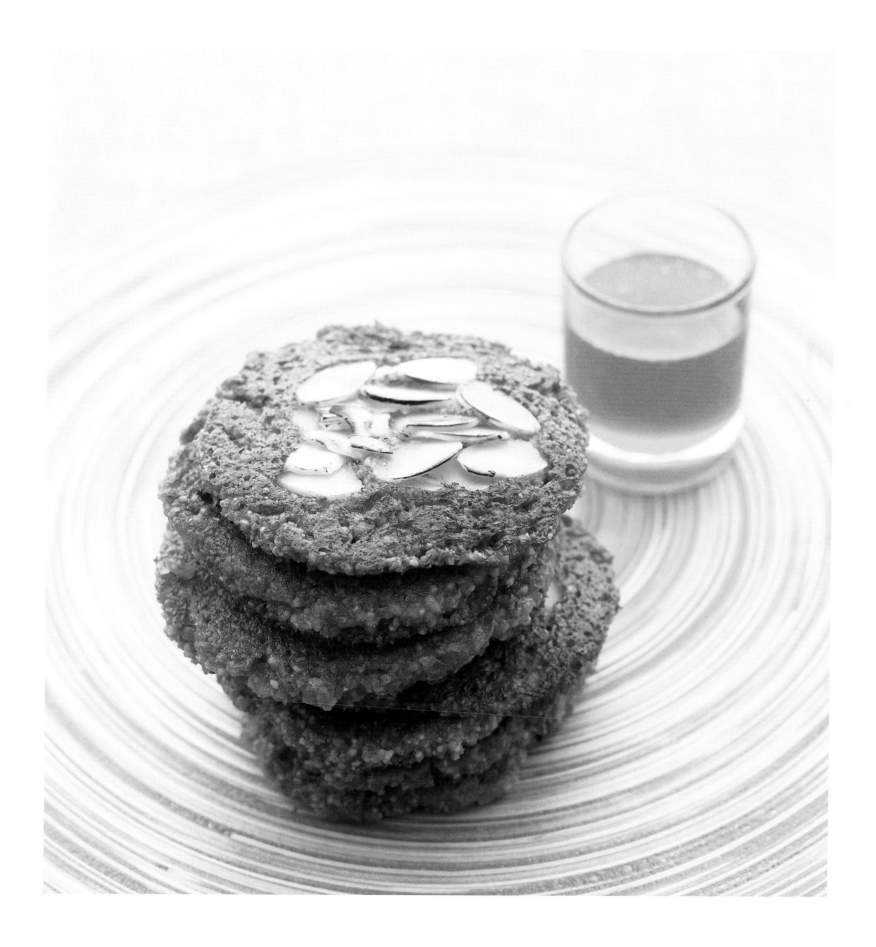

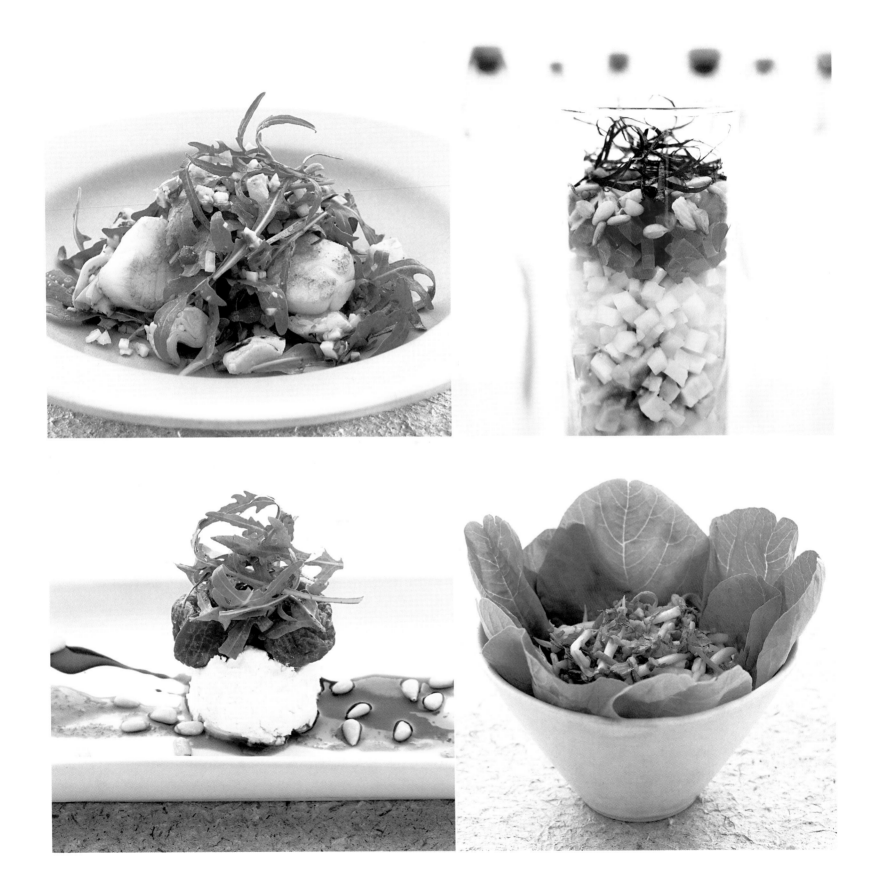

ZUCCHINI, ROCKET & SCALLOP SALAD Serves 2

SALAD
2 medium zucchinis, chopped
½ red onion, chopped
½ red capsicum, chopped
2 handfuls of rocket leaves
6 fresh scallops, shelled, without roe
2 ready roasted and marinated
artichokes, quartered
DRESSING
275 ml / 9¾ fl oz / 1⅛ cups extra virgin olive oil
90 ml / 3 fl oz / ⅓ cup lemon juice
2 small cloves garlic, minced
1 jalapeno chilli, chopped, add according
to taste
Small bunch coriander, chopped, add according
to taste
A large pinch of ground coriander seeds

DRESSING Combine all ingredients in a bowl and set aside. SALAD Marinate the zucchini, onion and red capsicum in the dressing for 3 hours. Sear scallops in a very hot non-stick pan (with the least amount of oil possible). Don't keep them in the pan too long, just seal them—as they are fresh they can be eaten slightly rare. Finally, toss the rocket with the dressed zucchini, onion and red capsicum and remove any surplus dressing. Place the salad on a plate and garnish with the seared scallops and roasted artichokes.

DETOX SALAD Serves 2

6 tomatoes, diced
5–6 stalks of celery with leaves, diced
2 avocados, diced
2 green apples, diced with skin
½ cucumber, diced with skin
Handful of dried seaweed torn into small pieces
4 tbsp almonds, toasted
4 tbsp pine nuts, toasted
Sprinkling of sunflower or linseeds
90 ml / 3 fl oz / ⅓ cup orange vinaigrette (see recipe on page 74)

Combine all ingredients in a salad bowl, pour over orange vinaigrette, mix thoroughly and serve.

GOAT'S CHEESE WITH TOMATO CONSERVE, TOMATO & ROCKET JUS Serves 2

TOMATO CONSERVE
4 beefsteak tomatoes, each weighing
about 400 g / 14 oz
Herbal salt substitute (see recipe on page 75),
to taste
2 lemons
4 tsp sugar
200 ml / 7 fl oz / ⅞ cup tomato juice
Tabasco sauce, to taste
ROCKET JUS
100 g / 3½ oz rocket
200 ml / 7 fl oz / 1 cup chilled olive oil
Herbal salt substitute (see recipe on page 75),
to taste
GOAT'S CHEESE
120 g (4¼ oz) goat's cheese
1 tbsp pine nuts, roasted
2 handfuls of rocket leaves

TOMATO CONSERVE Place tomatoes in a bowl of boiling water and leave for a few minutes, remove from water, peel the skin and take off the stems. Sprinkle with a little herbal salt. Wash lemons and rub the skin of one with some sugar. Arrange the lemon and tomatoes, stem side down, on a rack in a roasting pan. Rub the remaining sugar over the tomatoes and roast in the oven at 80°C / 176°F for 5–6 hours, or until the tomatoes are completely dehydrated and sugar frosted. Drain juice from the roasting pan into a saucepan and mix with tomato juice. Gently heat the mixture and reduce to a syrup. Season to taste with a few drops of Tabasco sauce and set aside. ROCKET JUS Clean the rocket thoroughly and remove the larger stalks. Blanch the leaves in well-salted boiling water, before cooling immediately in a bowl of iced water. Press or squeeze the water out of the greens with your hands. Purée the rocket in a blender, slowly adding the chilled olive oil until the purée holds together. You may not need all of the oil, and chilling it beforehand in the freezer will help bind the ingredients together. Rub the purée through a fine strainer, reserve the jus and season with herbal salt to taste. TO SERVE Spoon the goat's cheese in the middle of each plate and top with 2 pieces of tomato conserve. Toss the rocket leaves with a little of the tomato jus and place on the top of the tomato conserve. Drizzle rocket and tomato jus around the tower and serve with balsamic vinegar. To lighten the calorie load, a mixture of goat's cheese with cottage cheese can be used instead.

SIMPLE SPINACH SALAD Serves 2

3–4 handfuls of organic spinach, or as much as you can eat
1 carrot (or cucumber or capsicum), shredded
2–3 tbsp light soy sauce
3 tbsp lemon juice or cider vinegar
2 shallots, chopped
2 cloves garlic, chopped
1 carton alfalfa or 1 handful of bean sprouts
3 tbsp tahini

Immerse loose spinach in a bowl of cold water, rinse well and strain. On one side, mix half the shredded carrot (or cucumber or capsicum) with 2 tbsp soy sauce, 3 tbsp lemon juice or cider vinegar with chopped shallot and chopped garlic. Adjust the soy sauce and lemon juice to taste. Thin to desired consistency and toss the spinach in dressing. Now add the rest of the shredded carrots, sprouts, and any other vegetables of your choice. For more variation, a mixture of spinach and morning glory or rocket leaves can be used instead of just spinach.

OPPOSITE (CLOCKWISE FROM TOP LEFT): Zucchini, rocket and scallop salad; Detox salad; Simple spinach salad; Goat's cheese with tomato conserve, tomato and rocket jus.

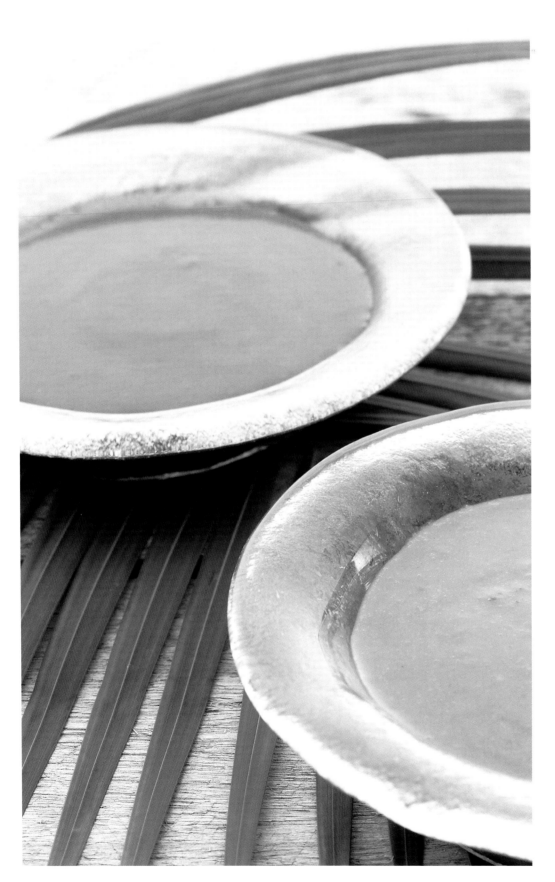

GAZPACHO SOUP Serves 2

700 ml / 1¼ pints / 3 cups tomato juice
1 tbsp extra virgin olive oil
1 tsp white wine vinegar
3 lime leaves
2 stalks of lemongrass
1 large red chilli
1 clove garlic, chopped
½ cucumber, peeled, deseeded and chopped
½ small red onion, chopped
½ green capsicum, deseeded and chopped
½ red capsicum, deseeded and chopped
Small bunch of coriander
½ tsp herbal salt substitute (see recipe on page 75)
¼ tsp ground black pepper

Place all ingredients in a food processor or blender and process until smooth. Transfer mixture to an airtight container, cover tightly and chill for at least 4 hours. Serve chilled.

CORN GAZPACHO SOUP
Serves 2

2 cobs of corn
425 ml / ¾ pint / 2 cups fresh tomato juice
1 tomato, diced
½ onion, chopped
½ red capsicum, diced
½ cucumber, diced
1 clove garlic, finely chopped
Small bunch fresh parsley, chopped
2 sprigs basil, leaves chopped
1 tsp lemon juice
½ tsp Worcestershire sauce
1 tbsp extra virgin olive oil
Herbal salt substitute (see recipe on page 75), to taste
Freshly ground black pepper, to taste

Boil the corn cobs for 5–10 minutes, scrape off the kernels and set aside. In a blender, combine tomato juice, tomato, onion, capsicum, cucumber, garlic, parsley and basil, blend on a high speed until puréed. Pour the contents of the blender into a glass bowl and stir in the corn and remaining ingredients. Transfer mixture to an airtight container, cover tightly and chill for at least 4 hours. Serve chilled.

Gazpacho soup; Corn gazpacho soup.
OPPOSITE (FROM TOP): Chilled vegetable soup; Roasted red capsicum soup.

CHILLED VEGETABLE SOUP
Serves 2

1 carrot, peeled and roughly chopped
1 stalk of celery, peeled and roughly chopped
½ small zucchini, roughly chopped
½ small red onion, chopped
½ red capsicum
Leaves of 2 large bok choi, sliced
Small bunch of coriander, chopped
Handful of green beans
Handful of mange tout
Handful of mungbean sprouts
Handful of sunflower sprouts
3 tbsp almonds, toasted and finely chopped
1 clove garlic, minced
1 tsp ginger juice, or 2 tsp minced ginger
1 tbsp sesame oil, or more, to taste
2 pieces of nori, cut into strips

Juice all ingredients in a durable juicer. Transfer mixture to an airtight container, cover tightly and chill for at least 4 hours. Serve chilled. The soup is especially refreshing when served cold. It can be served hot, but the ingredients will inevitably lose some goodness during the cooking process.

ROASTED RED CAPSICUM
SOUP Serves 2

5 red capsicums
½ tbsp olive oil
½ carrot, finely chopped
4–5 stalks of celery, finely chopped
1 large onion, chopped
Herbal salt substitute (see recipe on page 75), to taste
Freshly ground black pepper, to taste
1 L / 1¾ pints / 4 cups basic stock (see recipe on page 75)
1 small russet potato, peeled and sliced
1 bay leaf
Handful of fresh basil leaves

Place capsicums directly onto a lit hob. Once the skin is charred and blistered, remove from flame and scrape off the black skin. Set aside to cool. Heat olive oil in a large pan over a low heat. Add carrot, celery and onion, season lightly with herbal salt and pepper, and cook for 10 minutes. Add stock, potato and bay leaf and bring to a boil over a high heat. Lower the heat and simmer until the vegetables are completely tender. This will take about 15 minutes. Now the capsicums have cooled, take off the top, remove seeds and roughly chop, and add to the soup. Simmer for a further 10 minutes. Remove bay leaf and purée soup in a blender. Adjust the herbal salt and pepper to taste. TO SERVE Pour soup in warm bowls and sprinkle with chopped basil.

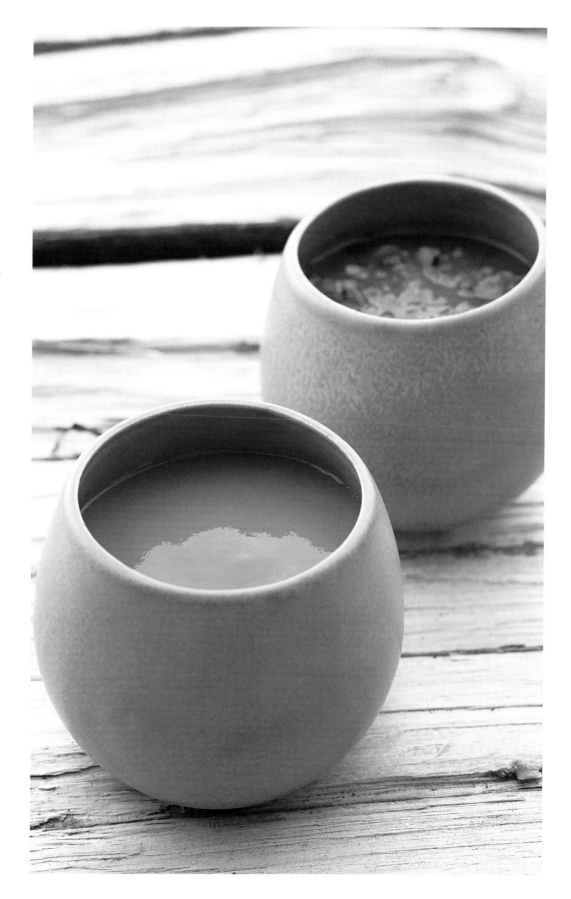

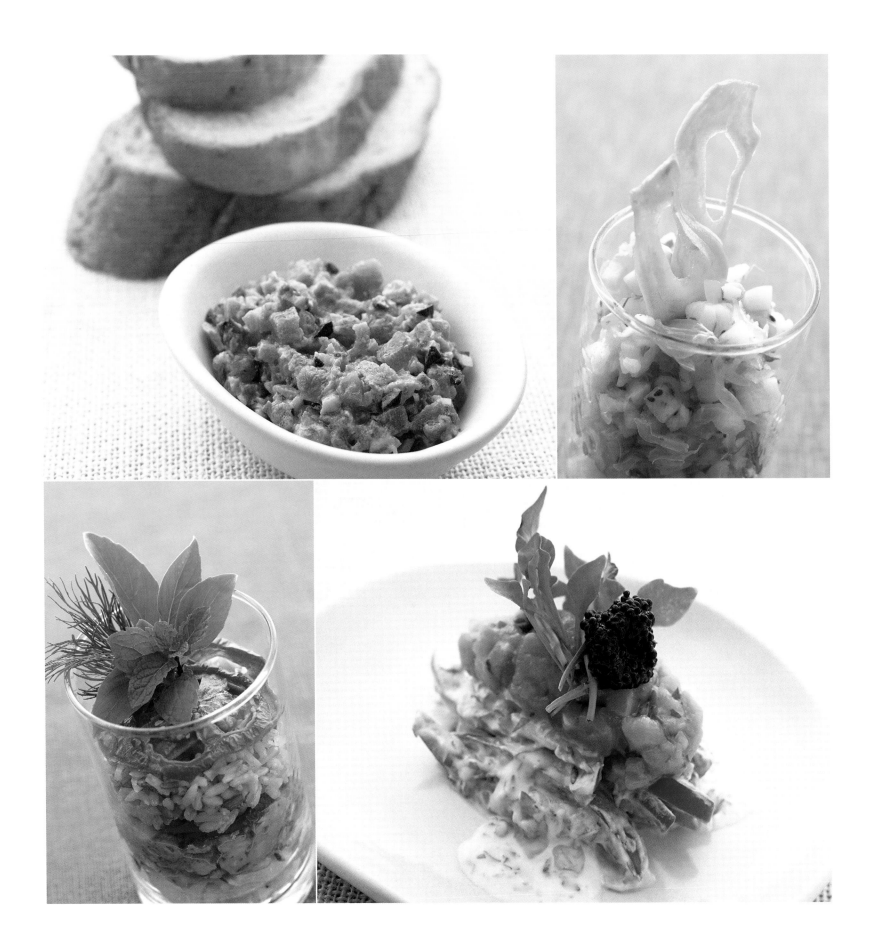

TUNA SANDWICH Serves 2

1 tin of tuna in brine
2 tsp extra virgin olive oil
1 shallot, finely chopped
2 tsp capers
1 tbsp chopped olives
2 gherkins, chopped
1 tsp English mustard

Drain tuna and mix with the olive oil, chopped shallot, capers, olives, gherkins and a dash of mustard. TO SERVE Sandwich between 2 slices of multigrain bread for each person and serve.

TIAN OF AVOCADO & WILD RICE Serves 2

AVOCADO
2 ripe avocados, mashed
2 small red onions, minced
2 small red capsicums, minced
Juice of ½ lime
1 tsp chopped coriander
1½ tsp kelp (sea seasoning)
A few sprigs of oregano
Cayenne pepper, to taste
WILD RICE
200 g / 7 oz wild rice
2 ready roasted and marinated artichokes, quartered
6 sun-dried tomatoes
½ an iceberg lettuce
Small handful of herbal mesclun
4 tbsp tomato dressing (see recipe on page 74)
1 tbsp pesto (see recipe on page 75)

AVOCADO Combine all ingredients in a bowl and set aside. WILD RICE Soak wild rice in cold water for 3 days, changing the water daily. TO SERVE Layer the avocado mash with the lettuce, artichoke, wild rice and sun-dried tomatoes in a tall glass. Garnish with the herbal mesclun and serve with the tomato dressing and pesto.

SEAFOOD & TROPICAL FRUIT CEVICHE Serves 2

80 g / 2¾ oz mixed seafood (prawns, scallops, sea bass), diced
60 g / 2¼ oz pomelo, segmented and shredded
1 green apple, diced
1 red apple, diced
1 dragonfruit, diced
1 ripe mango, diced
2 large red chillies
2 shallots, chopped
Large bunch of coriander, chopped
4 tbsp extra virgin olive oil
Dash of lime juice
Herbal salt substitute (see recipe on page 75), to taste
Freshly ground black pepper, to taste

Place seafood in a steamer and steam for about 30 seconds. Combine all ingredients into a large bowl and season. Chill in the refrigerator for 3–4 hours. TO SERVE Place in a glass and garnish with fresh herbs.

TARTARE OF WILD SALMON WITH SPICED YOGHURT RELISH Serves 2

300 g / 10½ oz wild salmon
1 shallot, finely chopped
2 tsp spicy green mustard
2 tsp extra virgin olive oil
1 tsp lime juice
Herbal salt substitute (see recipe on page 75), to taste
Freshly ground black pepper, to taste
6 tbsp spiced yoghurt relish (see recipe on page 75)
2 tsp seaweed caviar (available in Japanese supermarkets)
Handful of watercress
Few drops of truffle oil

Mince salmon with the finely chopped shallots, spicy green mustard, olive oil, lime juice, herbal salt and pepper, and set aside. TO SERVE Spoon the spiced yoghurt relish onto the middle of a plate and pile the salmon tartar on top. Complete the stack with watercress and seaweed caviar; drizzle a little truffle oil around the salmon and serve immediately.

OPPOSITE (CLOCKWISE FROM TOP LEFT): Tuna sandwich; Seafood and tropical fruit ceviche; Tartare of wild salmon with spiced yoghurt relish; Tian of avocado and wild rice.

CHARGRILLED TUNA Serves 2

300 g / 10½ oz ocean tuna
6 tbsp salsa verde (see recipe on page 75)
4 sheets of nori
2 tsp herbal salt substitute (see recipe on page 75)
1 tsp chilli powder
1 butterhead lettuce, or a large handful of rocket or mizuna
3 tsp extra virgin olive oil mixed with 1 tsp balsamic vinegar

Rub the tuna with the salsa and leave to marinate for 20 minutes. Once ready, grill the tuna (preferably under an open flame) until seared on the outside and still quite rare inside. Break the nori into small pieces and season with herbal salt and chilli powder, then mix with salad leaves and set aside. To enhance flavour, sprinkle the salad with a few drops of extra virgin olive oil and balsamic vinegar. TO SERVE Place tuna in the middle of each plate, decorate with the salad and drizzle around the remaining salsa. Serve with brown or wild rice if desired.

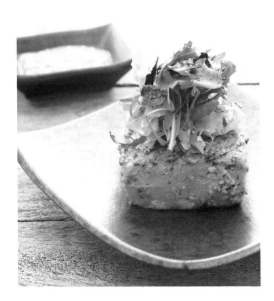

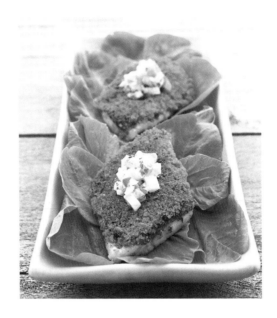

CHERMOULAH SPICED SEA BASS ON AN ORGANIC SPINACH SALAD Serves 2

CHERMOULAH SPICED SEA BASS
6 tbsp dry chermoulah spice (see recipe on page 74)
2 sea bass (or other lean fish) fillets with skin, each weighing about 150 g / 5½ oz
2 tsp vegetable oil
ORGANIC SPINACH SALAD
4 handfuls of wild spinach
2 tbsp mustard dressing (see recipe on page 74)
6 tbsp spiced yoghurt relish (see recipe on page 75)

CHERMOULAH SPICED SEA BASS
Preheat the oven to 180°C / 360°F. Rub chermoulah spice onto the skin of the sea bass fillets and marinate for 30 minutes. In a non-stick frying-pan, heat vegetable oil, and sear fish, skin side down, until the spice crust becomes crispy. Flip over and sear on the flesh side. Next place the fish, skin side down, on a slightly oiled tray and transfer to the preheated oven. Bake fish for about 2–3 minutes until cooked. ORGANIC SPINACH SALAD Toss the washed and wilted spinach leaves with the mustard dressing and pepper. For some variety, crunchy chopped green vegetables can also be added. TO SERVE Dress the plate with salad and place the fish on top. Serve with spiced yoghurt relish on the side.

STEAMED SALMON WITH SOY, GINGER & CHINESE BLACK MUSHROOMS Serves 2

4½ tbsp basic stock (see recipe on page 75)
2½ tbsp sesame oil
2 tbsp oyster sauce
2 tsp dark soy sauce
2 tsp wild honey
2 salmon fillets, each weighing about 175 g / 6 oz
1 thumb-size piece of young ginger, sliced
6 spring onions, halved lengthwise
6 wood ear mushrooms, sliced
1 large bunch of coriander

Whisk stock, sesame oil, oyster sauce, dark soy sauce and honey together and taste for flavour. Place salmon in a stainless steel bowl, layer the top and bottom of the fish with slices of young ginger and spring onion. Next, pour over enough sauce to submerge half of the salmon. Add wood ear mushroom and cover the bowl with cling film. Next place the bowl in a steaming tray, covering the tray tightly with a lid, and steam over boiling water for 20–25 minutes. TO SERVE Once ready, serve immediately with steamed brown rice, or a mix of white and wild rice, and garnish with coriander.

Chargrilled tuna; Chermoulah spiced sea bass on an organic spinach salad.
OPPOSITE: Steamed salmon with soy, ginger and Chinese black mushrooms.

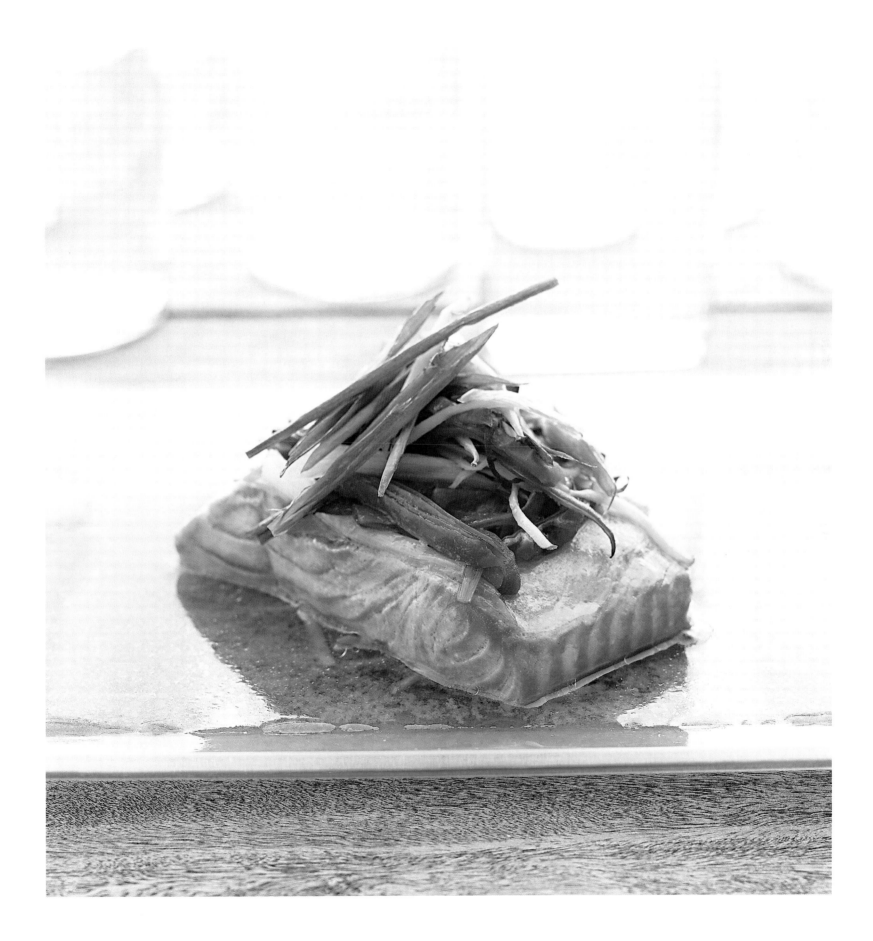

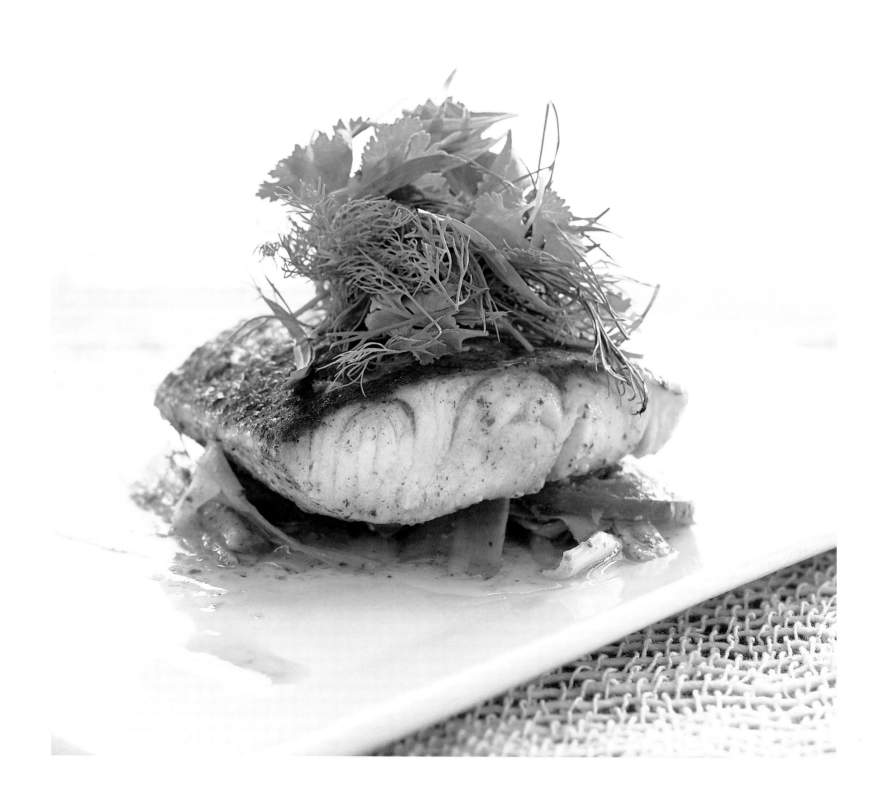

ROASTED BARRACUDA Serves 2

2 tbsp fresh orange juice
4 tbsp fresh lime juice
A pinch of grated orange zest
A pinch of grated lime zest
2 shallots or ¼ red onion, chopped
1 tbsp olive oil or canola oil
2 barracuda (or white snapper, grouper, or sea bass) fillets, each weighing about 150 g / 5½ oz
1 clove garlic, roughly chopped
A large pinch of chopped fresh basil
A large pinch of chopped fresh mint
A pinch of fresh thyme leaves
A pinch of herbal salt substitute (see recipe on page 75)
A pinch of coarsely ground black pepper
½ leek, including tender green top, halved lengthwise and sliced into 4 cm / 1½ inch slices
1 large tomato, sliced into 1 cm / ½ inch slices
mixed salad leaves

To prepare marinade, combine orange and lime juice, orange and lime zest, shallots and ½ tbsp of olive or canola oil in a shallow baking dish. Next, score the skin of the fish in a diamond pattern and place in the marinade, turning once to coat. Cover the dish and refrigerate for 30 minutes, turning the fish occasionally. Preheat the oven to 225°C / 430°F and lightly coat another shallow baking dish with cooking spray. In a blender, combine garlic, basil, mint, thyme, the remaining olive oil, and half of the herbal salt and pepper, and blend to a purée. In a small bowl, combine half of the herb purée with chopped leek and gently toss. Spread the leek mixture evenly over the bottom of the prepared baking dish and top with a single layer of tomato slices. Sprinkle with remaining herbal salt and pepper. Remove fish from marinade, pat dry and discard unused marinade. Rub remaining herb purée over the fish, coating both sides, and place on top of the tomatoes. Cover the dish tightly with aluminium foil and place in oven for 10 minutes, uncover and roast for another 5 minutes. Feel the fish throughout; it should be opaque when tested with the tip of a knife. TO SERVE Divide vegetables between warmed plates, pile fish on top and serve with mixed salad leaves.

CRUNCHY WHITE SNAPPER WITH A PISTACHIO, MACADAMIA & COCONUT CRUST Serves 2

60 g / 2¼ oz fresh multi-grain breadcrumbs
2 tbsp mixture of ground pistachio nuts, macadamia nuts and desiccated coconut
A large pinch of chopped coriander
½ tsp grated lemon zest
½ tsp herbal salt substitute (see recipe on page 75)
2 tbsp skimmed milk
2 fillets of white snapper, each weighing about 150 g / 5½ oz
¼ tsp ground black pepper
4 tbsp white truffle oil
3–4 handfuls of salad leaves (or enough for 2 people)

Preheat oven to 230°C / 440°F. Place a small wire rack in a shallow non-stick roasting pan. On a shallow-rimmed plate, combine breadcrumbs, nut mixture, coriander, lemon zest and half of the herbal salt. Pour milk into a shallow bowl and dip each fish fillet in the milk. Then dredge fish with the nut mixture, coating each fillet completely and pressing lightly so the mixture sticks to the fish. Place fillets on the rack in the roasting pan, making sure that they don't touch, and sprinkle evenly with the remaining herbal salt and pepper. Transfer to the oven and bake for 10–12 minutes, until the fish is opaque throughout when tested with the tip of a knife and the crust is golden brown. TO SERVE Transfer to warmed plates, drizzle with a little truffle oil and serve with mixed salad leaves.

Crunchy white snapper with a pistachio, macadamia and coconut crust.
OPPOSITE: Roasted barracuda.

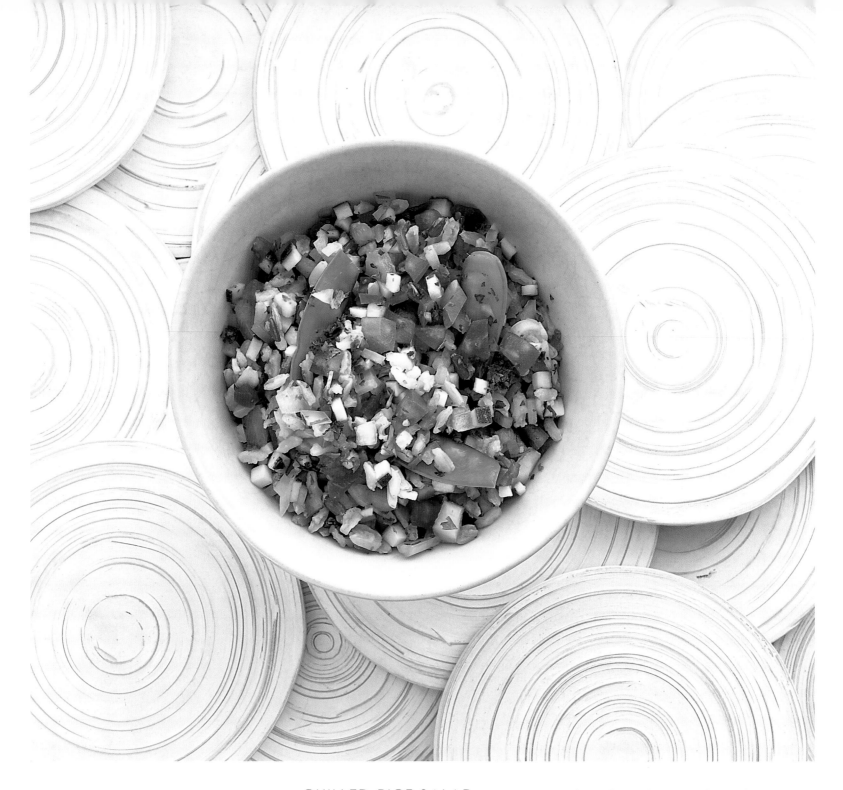

CHILLED RICE SALAD Serves 2

2 handfuls of wild rice
200 g / 7 oz green peas, boiled for 3–4 minutes
6 onions, finely chopped
2 stalks of celery, finely chopped
1 green capsicum, finely chopped
1 large tomato, finely chopped
1 small zucchini, finely chopped
1–2 tbsp chopped jalapeno chilli
¼ tsp mustard powder
Small handful of parsley, chopped
A pinch of chopped tarragon
125 ml / 4 fl oz / ½ cup cider or white
wine vinegar
Lettuce, any kind

Soak wild rice in a bowl of water for three days, changing the water daily. When ready, mix rice with the rest of the ingredients and chill in the refrigerator. TO SERVE Spoon rice salad on a bed of crunchy mixed lettuce.

Chilled rice salad.
OPPOSITE: Mediterranean
pasta.

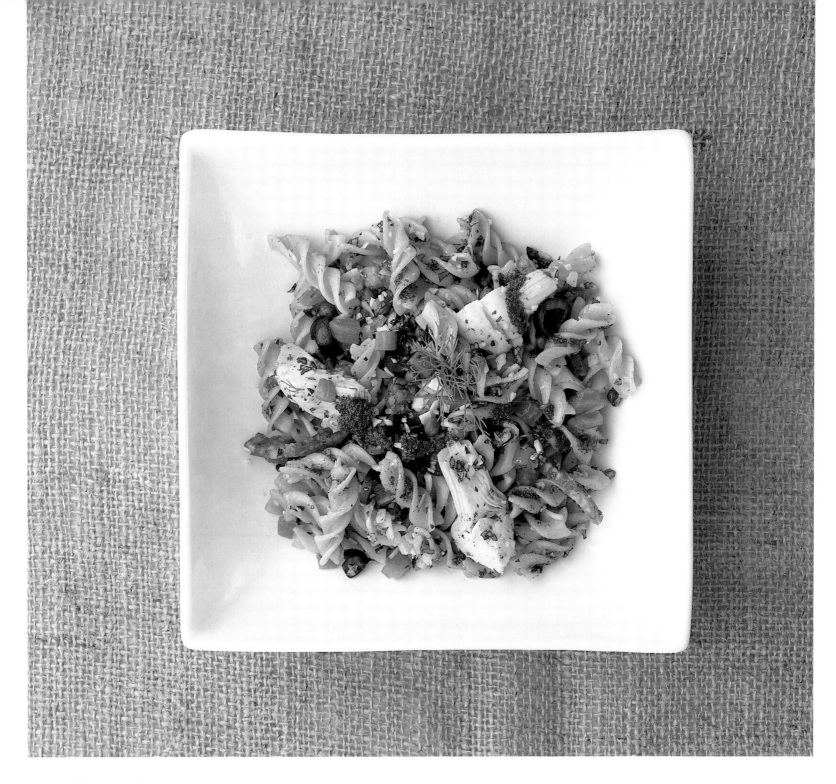

MEDITERRANEAN PASTA
Serves 2

250 g / 9 oz wholewheat pasta
1 tbsp olive oil
1 clove garlic, minced
2 tbsp white wine
2 tbsp pitted calamata olives, sliced into thirds
1½ tbsp chopped almonds, with skins
1 tbsp chopped shallot
1 tbsp capers
5–6 sun-dried tomatoes, chopped
2 ready roasted and marinated artichokes, quartered
A large pinch of chopped basil
A pinch of freshly ground black pepper

Cook pasta in boiling water for 8–10 minutes, or until al dente. In a medium saucepan, heat olive oil and add garlic. Cook on a low heat for 3–4 minutes, add remaining ingredients and cook for another 5–10 minutes. Add the pasta and mix well. Cook for another 2–3 minutes, before serving. For a meaty alternative, add 2 tbsp of chorizo, pepperoni or salami (julienne).

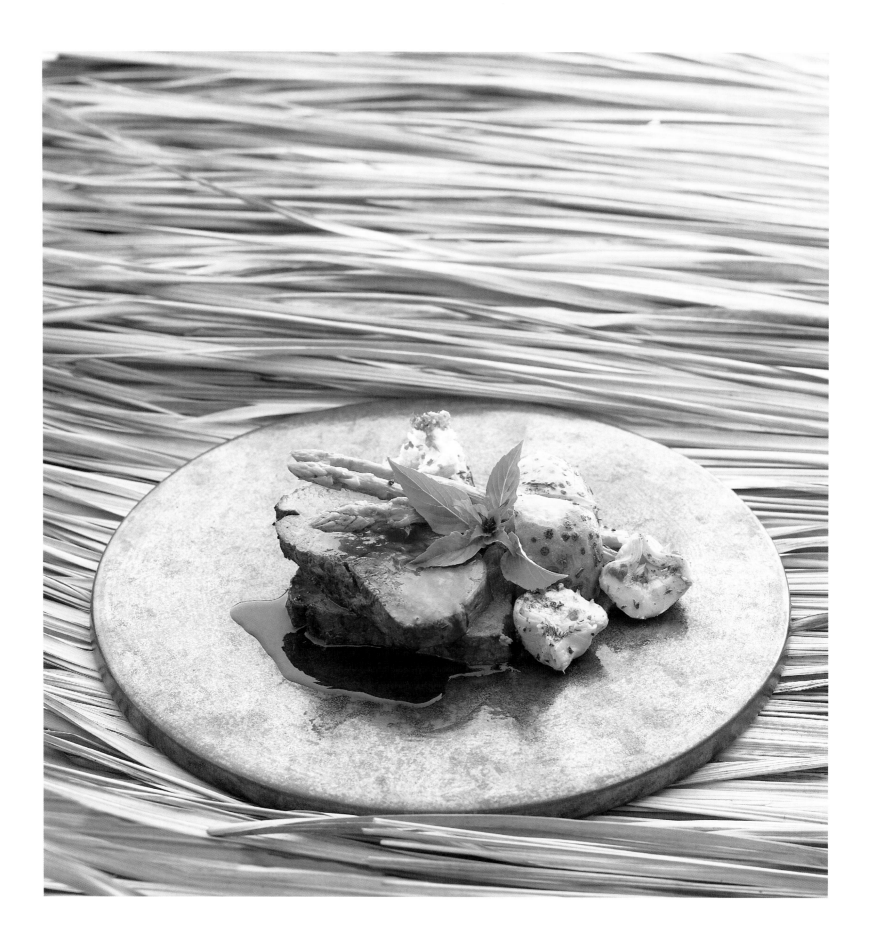

ROAST BEEF WITH ALL THE TRIMMINGS Serves 2

ROAST BEEF
700 g / 1 lb 9 oz beef sirloin or striploin
1 tbsp herbal salt substitute (see recipe on page 75)
1½ tbsp mustard (Dijon, English or spicy green)
A large pinch of freshly ground black pepper
1 tsp rosemary, chopped
1 tsp thyme, chopped
GRAVY
175 g / 6 oz celeriac, peeled and chopped
1 shallot, sliced
1 carrot, diced
1 leek, roughly chopped
2 tbsp red wine, optional
1 tsp Dijon mustard
1 tsp wholegrain mustard
Herbal salt substitute, to taste
Freshly ground black pepper to taste
A large pinch of chopped tarragon
1 tbsp flour mixed with 1 tbsp butter
TRIMMINGS
4 medium or 8 small new potatoes
1 tbsp dry chermoulah spice (see recipe on page 74)
5 tbsp extra vifrgin olive oil
2 carrots, chopped into chunks
2 red capsicums, roughly chopped
2 zucchinis, chopped into chunks
1 medium eggplant, chopped into chunks
small bunch of herbs (thyme, basil, rosemary and oregano), chopped
2 cloves garlic
4 tbsp low-fat ricotta or cottage cheese or mustard dressing (see recipe on page 74)
Parsley to garnish

ROAST BEEF Preheat oven to 180°C / 360°F. Score the fat on the beef and rub with herbal salt, mustard, pepper, rosemary and thyme. Place on a roasting pan and roast for 75 minutes. When meat is ready, it should be pink in colour and at 52°C / 125°F on a thermometer, remove from the oven and rest for up to 1 hour, 30 minutes at least, in a warm place to ensure the temperature distributes evenly across the meat. GRAVY While meat is resting, pour juice from the roasting pan into a bowl. Transfer to the freezer to 'shock chill'; this will bring the fat to the top in a hard, solid paste (be careful not to freeze the gravy). Scoop off the fat and sieve remaining gravy into another bowl. In a frying-pan sauté celeriac, shallot, carrot, and leek until glazed. Add wine, if using, then gravy and reduce to required thickness over a high heat. Add mustard and adjust seasoning. To finish, strain gravy and add tarragon. If the gravy is too thin, quickly stir in 1 tsp of the flour/butter mixture. TRIMMINGS Scrub potatoes clean, leaving the skin on. Rub the dry chermoulah spice onto potatoes and place on a sheet of aluminium foil. Sprinkle over 2 tbsp of the olive oil. Wrap foil around each potato and roast for 35–40 minutes. Large potatoes may take up to 50 minutes. In a

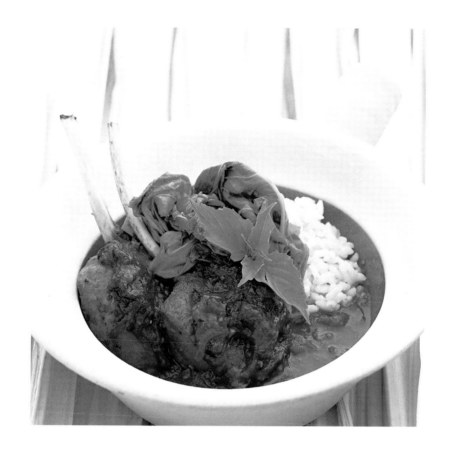

separate baking dish, coat vegetables, chopped herbs and garlic in remaining olive oil and roast in the oven with potatoes for 30–35 minutes. TO SERVE Once potatoes are ready, remove the foil, cut in the middle and top with low-fat ricotta or cottage cheese, or mustard dressing and garnish with parsley. Serve with beef, vegetables and gravy.

LAMB OSSO-BUCCO WITH THAI HERBS Serves 2

LAMB OSSO-BUCCO
180 g / 6 oz shallots, sliced
2 tsp sesame oil
440 ml / 16 fl oz / 2⅛ cups tamarind juice
6–8 tbsp hoi sin sauce
Juice of 1 small pomelo
6 tbsp wild honey
2–3 tbsp Worcestershire sauce
2 tbsp Dijon mustard
5 ginger flowers, chopped (optional)
4 long stalks of lemongrass, chopped
Thumb-size piece of young ginger, chopped
2 cloves garlic, chopped
6 lamb cutlets
ACCOMPANIMENTS
150 g / 5½ oz arborio rice
1 L / 1¾ pints / 4 cups warm basic stock (see recipe on page 75)
4 handfuls of spinach

LAMB OSSO-BUCCO Preheat the oven to 220°C / 430°F. To prepare the marinade, place shallots in a saucepan and sauté over a medium heat with sesame oil. Once fragrant, turn to a low heat and add tamarind juice, hoi sin sauce, pomelo juice, honey, Worcestershire sauce, Dijon mustard, ginger flowers, lemongrass, young ginger and garlic and bring to a boil. Simmer until sauce thickens. Set aside to cool. Season lamb cutlets. Place a shallow pan over a high heat, once it is smoking hot, sear lamb quickly for 2 minutes on each side. Place lamb cutlets in a roasting pan and pour over marinade. Roast at 220°C / 430°F for approximately 7–9 minutes. ACCOMPANIMENTS While lamb is roasting, place risotto rice into a heavy-based pan and stir in 1 ladle of stock, once absorbed repeat until all stock is used up. Rice should be creamy with a little nuttiness. Quickly sauté the spinach. TO SERVE Place 3 lamb cutlets on each plate, pour over a good helping of the leftover marinade sauce, and serve with risotto and sautéed spinach.

Lamb osso-bucco with Thai herbs.
OPPOSITE: Roast beef with all the trimmings.

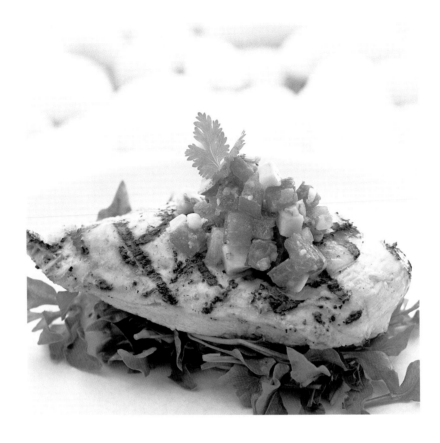

GRILLED CHICKEN WITH TOMATO-AVOCADO SALSA Serves 2

TOMATO-AVOCADO SALSA
¼ avocado
2–3 tbsp fresh lime juice
2 ripe plum tomatoes, chopped, or 6 cherry tomatoes, halved
¼ small red onion, finely chopped
½ jalapeño chilli, seeded and diced
1 tbsp chopped fresh coriander
GRILLED CHICKEN
2–3 tbsp low-fat yoghurt
¼ small red onion
2 tbsp fresh lime juice
Small handful of fresh coriander
2 boneless and skinless free range chicken breasts, each weighing about 175 g / 6 oz
A pinch of freshly ground black pepper

SALSA Chop the avocado and sprinkle it with 2 tbsp of lime juice to keep it from browning. In a small bowl, combine tomatoes, red onion, jalapeño chilli and coriander. Add the avocado and remaining lime juice to the bowl and toss to combine. This can be made in advance and stored in the refrigerator for up to one day. GRILLED CHICKEN In a food processor, purée the yoghurt, red onion, lime juice and coriander to make a yoghurt marinade. Transfer marinade to a shallow bowl or a plastic bag. Add the chicken and coat well with the marinade. Refrigerate for a minimum of 1 hour, or up to 8 hours. Preheat the grill to medium-high. Remove the chicken and discard any remaining marinade. Season the chicken with black pepper. Grill on both sides until cooked through (about 6 minutes per side). TO SERVE Place grilled chicken breast on the centre of each plate and top with tomato-avocado salsa.

WOK-FRIED CHICKEN WITH GINGER & SESAME Serves 2

CHICKEN
2 tsp sesame oil
2 tsp cornflour
Freshly ground black pepper, to taste
Large thumb-size piece of ginger, julienne
2 free-range chicken breasts, each weighing about 175 g / 6 oz, sliced
STIR-FRY
3 tbsp sesame oil
2 tbsp abalone sauce
2 tsp Chinese rice wine or sake or dry vermouth
2 tsp wild honey
2 tsp oyster sauce
1 tsp light soy sauce
1 tsp dark soy sauce
35 g spring onion, chopped
Herbal salt substitute (see recipe on page 75), to taste
Freshly ground black pepper, to taste

CHICKEN Combine sesame oil, cornflour, black pepper and ginger. Transfer to a bowl with sliced chicken. Marinate for at least 1 hour. Then blanch chicken for 1½ minutes, cool the chicken in iced-water and set aside. STIR-FRY Heat wok over a high heat, add sesame oil followed by blanched chicken. Stir-fry for a few minutes away from heat. Return to heat and add all stir-fry ingredients, stirring continuously. Season to taste. TO SERVE Serve with a mix of steamed white and wild rice.

Grilled chicken with tomato-avocado salsa.
OPPOSITE: Wok-fried chicken with ginger & sesame.

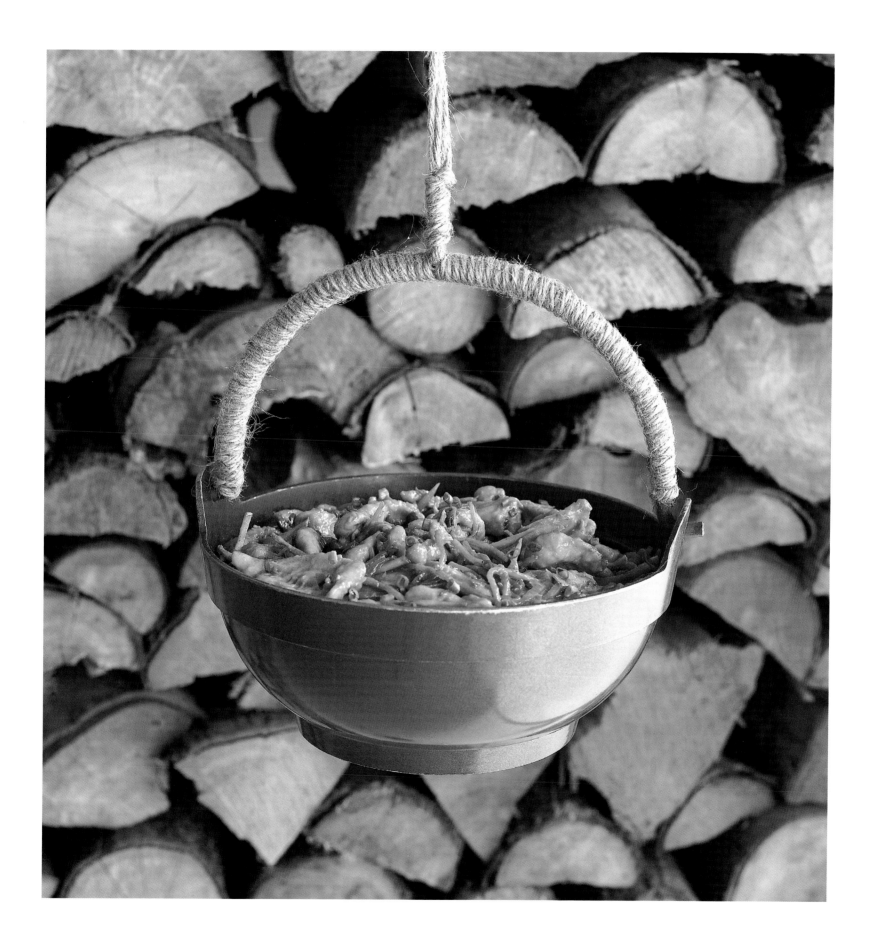

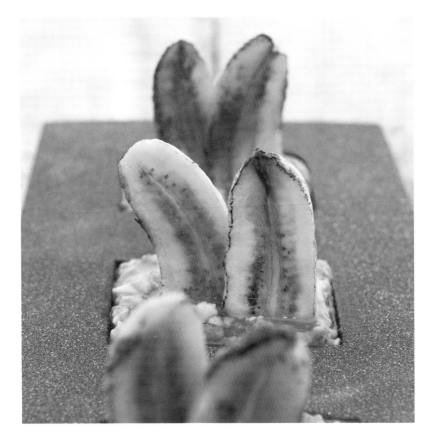

TIAN OF BANANAS WITH NUTS & RAISINS Serves 2

SAUCE
1 tsp butter
½ tbsp brown sugar
1 tsp wild honey
1 tsp walnut oil
1 tbsp low-fat milk
A pinch of cinnamon powder
½ tbsp dark or golden raisins
BANANAS
2 large bananas
1½ tbsp mixed chopped nuts (almonds, Brazil nuts and walnuts)
½ tsp canola oil
1 tbsp dark rum (or use unsweetened apple juice if preferred)

SAUCE Melt butter in a heavy-based pan. Stir in brown sugar, wild honey and walnut oil. Continue to stir until sugar has completely dissolved, about 3 minutes. Stir in milk, bit by bit, followed by cinnamon powder and simmer, stirring continuously, until the sauce thickens slightly (about another 3 minutes). Remove from heat and stir in raisins. Set aside and keep warm. BANANAS Peel bananas, and cut each crosswise into 3 sections. Cut each section in half lengthwise. Lightly coat a large non-stick frying-pan with canola oil and place over medium-high heat. Add bananas and sauté until they start to brown (3–4 minutes). Transfer to a plate and keep warm. Add rum to the pan, bring to the boil and deglaze the pan, stirring with a wooden spoon to scrape up any browned banana from the bottom of the pan. Cook until reduced by half, about 30–45 seconds. Return bananas to the pan to warm up again. TO SERVE Divide bananas among plates, in neat stacks. Drizzle with the warm sauce and serve.

APPLE CRUMBLE Makes 8 servings

SPICE MIX
Small thumb-size piece ginger, grated
1 tbsp cinnamon powder
2 tsp cardamom pods
1 tsp cloves
1 tsp coriander seeds
APPLE CRUMBLE
6 green apples, peeled, seeded and sliced
Juice of 1 lemon
60 g / 2¼ oz wholemeal flour
40 g / 1½ oz dark brown sugar
2 tbsp margarine, cut into thin slices
40 g / 1½ oz rolled oats

SPICE MIX Grind all ingredients together and keep in a screw-top jar. APPLE CRUMBLE Preheat oven to 190°C / 375°F. Use a 23 cm (9 in) round pie mould and grease with a little butter. Arrange apple slices around the base of the dish. Sprinkle with lemon juice and 1 tsp spice mix. In a small bowl, mix flour and brown sugar. Next, crumble the margarine into the flour-sugar mixture; use your hands to do this. Add the oats and mix thoroughly. Sprinkle flour mixture on top of the apple. Bake until apples are soft and the topping is browned (about 30 minutes). TO SERVE Cut into 8 even slices and serve warm with a spoon of low-fat natural yoghurt if desired.

Tian of bananas with nuts & raisins.
OPPOSITE: Apple crumble.

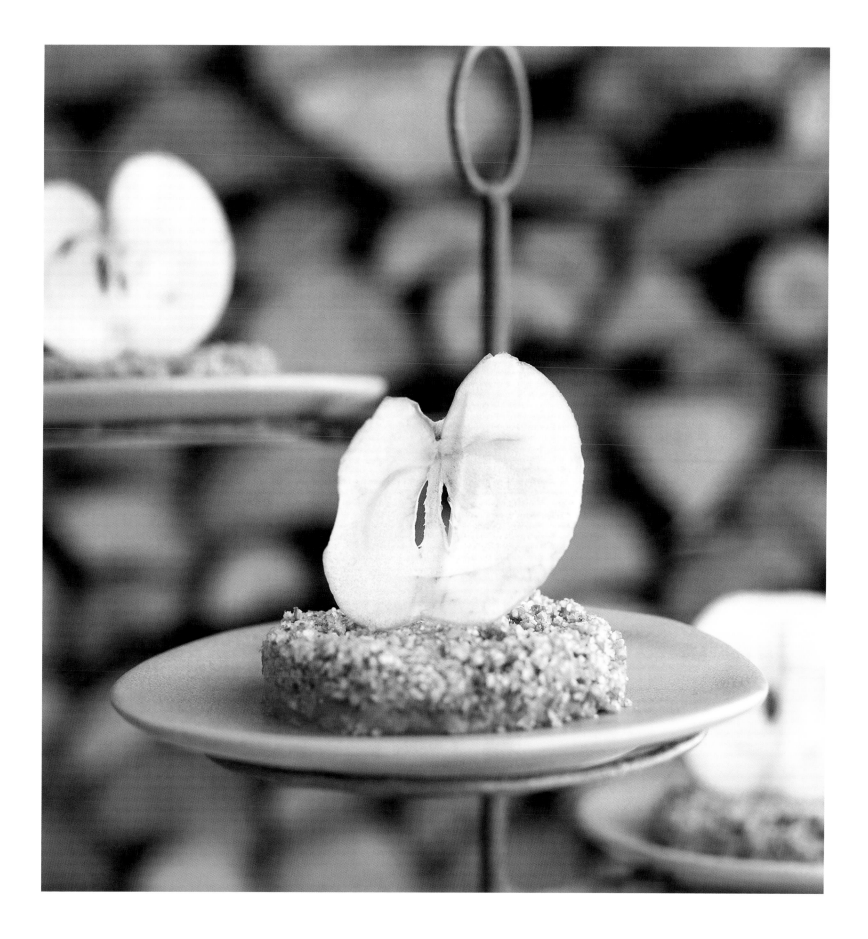

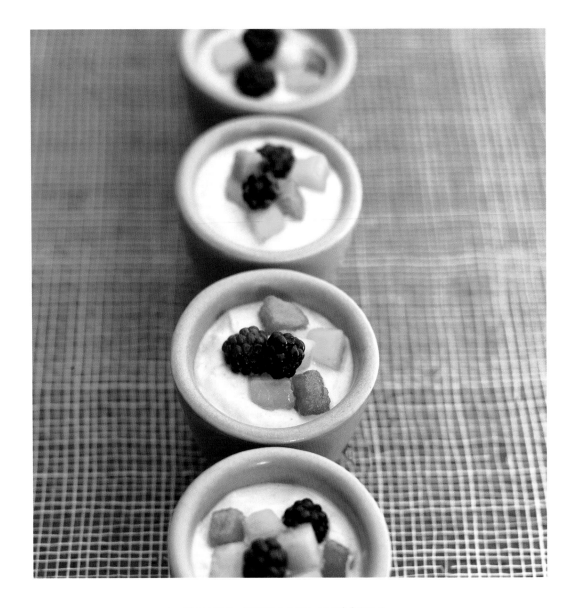

A QUICK CREAMY DESSERT
Serves 2

85 g / 3 oz low-fat cottage cheese
85 g / 3 oz low-fat natural yoghurt
3 tbsp wild honey
1 tbsp Amaretto liqueur (or Crème de Cassis)
A large pinch of fresh chopped herbs such as
lemongrass, kaffir lime leaves, lavender or grated
lime zest
375 g / 13 oz fresh fruit, combination of berries
(strawberries, blueberries, blackberries), with
mango, banana, melon or peach, diced

In a small bowl, whisk together cottage cheese,
natural yoghurt, wild honey, liqueur and herbs. In a
larger bowl, combine the diced fruit and cottage
cheese/yoghurt mixture. Stir gently to mix. Cover
and refrigerate until well chilled (about 1 hour).
TO SERVE Divide between 2 glasses and garnish
with some more fresh fruit.

A quick creamy dessert.
OPPOSITE: Balsamic marinated
fruit with vanilla and mint.

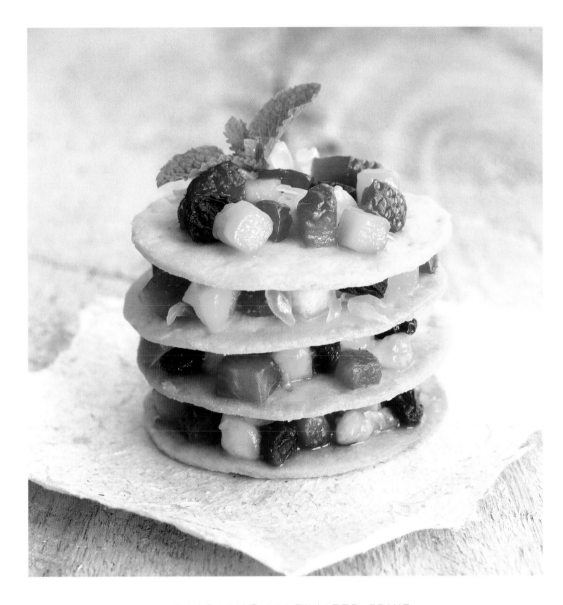

BALSAMIC MARINATED FRUIT
WITH VANILLA & MINT Serves 2

4 tbsp balsamic vinegar
2 tbsp brown sugar
A pinch of chopped mint leaves
Seeds from 2 vanilla pods
300 g / 10½ oz mixed fruit such as
strawberries, raspberries, blueberries,
blackcurrants, mango, banana
8 shortbread biscuits

In a small bowl, whisk together the balsamic
vinegar, brown sugar, chopped mint and vanilla
seeds. In another bowl, mix the fruit and pour
the balsamic vinegar mixture over the fruit.
Leave to marinate for 10–15 minutes. Drain the
marinade. Refrigerate or serve immediately. TO
SERVE Layer fruit with the shortbread biscuits.

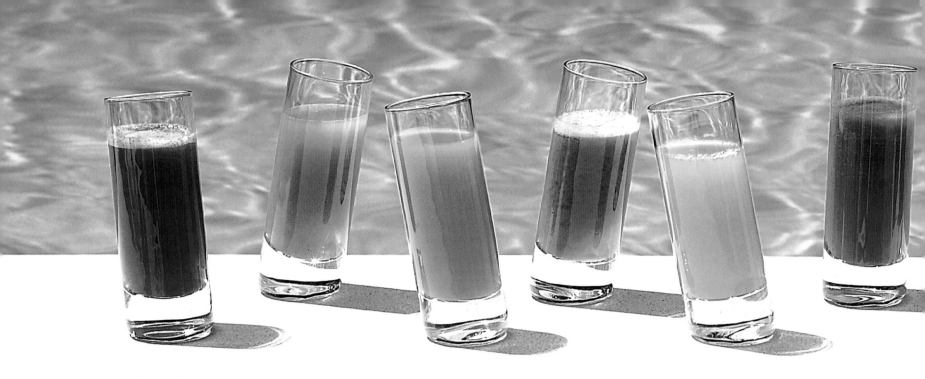

BEETROOT SPRITZER*

120 ml / 4 fl oz / ½ cup beetroot juice
150 ml / 5 fl oz / ⅔ cup soda
2 tbsp lime juice
Mix juices, pour into tall glasses and serve.

CARROT, CITRUS AND GINGER JUICE*

1 lime peeled and chopped
4 large carrots, juiced
Juice of ¼ pomelo
Juice of 3 oranges, preferably navel oranges
2.5 cm / 1 inch slice ginger
Zest of 1 lime
Using a blender, blend all ingredients together until smooth and serve.

CLEANSING JUICE*

2 medium beetroots, raw
Small handful of fresh parsley
2 green apples
Handful of wheatgrass, pressed (leave out if unavailable)
4 tsp wild honey, optional
Ice
Using a blender, blend ingredients together until smooth, adding ice to desired consistency, and serve.

ENERGIZER

4 carrots, scrubbed well or peeled
1 green apple
2 stalks of celery
3 red kale leaves
¼ inch ginger root
½ fennel bulb
Process all ingredients in a blender until creamy and serve.

An array of fresh tangy and revitalizing juices.
OPPOSITE: Natural ingredients for teas that will improve health and well-being.

GREEN VITAMIN BOOSTER

120 g / 4¼ oz baby spinach
1 green capsicum
5–7 stalks of celery
100 g / 3½ oz celery leaves
120 g / 4½ oz rocket leaves
100 g / 3½ oz butterhead or iceberg lettuce
Small bunch of coriander
Freshly ground black pepper or Tabasco, to taste
Using a blender, blend all ingredients together until smooth and serve.

MEMORY ENHANCER

4–5 carrots
3 stalks of celery with leaves
¼ head of a small cabbage, cut into sections
¼ lemon (peeled if not organic)
Cut off the green tops of the carrots and scrub well, no need to peel them. Wash the celery and cabbage and juice them with carrots. Add lemon to taste and serve.

PINEAPPLE AND GINGER ENERGY BOOSTER*

200 ml / 7 fl oz / ⅞ cup unsweetened pineapple juice
A pinch of chopped fresh mint
1 cm / ½ inch slice of ginger
Using a blender, blend all ingredients together until smooth and serve.

REJUVENATOR*

2 green apples
1 cucumber
4 sticks of celery
1 fennel bulb
2 handfuls of spinach
1 handful of parsley
Juice of ¼ pomelo (if unavailable, juice of ½ grapefruit)
Combine ingredients in a juicer and serve.

SALAD IN A GLASS*

3 cucumbers, juiced
4 green apples, juiced
5–7 stalks of celery, juiced
2 ripe tomatoes
Large bunch of parsley, juiced
½ iceberg lettuce, juiced
Using a blender, blend all ingredients together until smooth and serve.

SUMMER MINT MAGIC

1 pineapple
2 green apples
Handful of mint leaves
Remove the skin from the pineapple and cut into chunks. Juice all ingredients in a juicer, pour into tall glasses and serve.

TOMATO AND WHEATGRASS SHOOTER*

10 medium tomatoes, juiced
5–7 stalks of celery, juiced
2 handfuls of wheatgrass, pressed
½ tsp Worcestershire sauce
Blend ingredients together until smooth and serve.

V8*

2 handfuls of spinach
6 stalks of celery
4 asparagus stalks
2 large tomatoes
2 cherry tomatoes to garnish
Bunch spinach with celery and pass through a juicer. Juice asparagus with large tomatoes. Mix juices into tall glasses, garnish with a cherry tomatoes and serve.

* denotes those juices that are suitable for detox

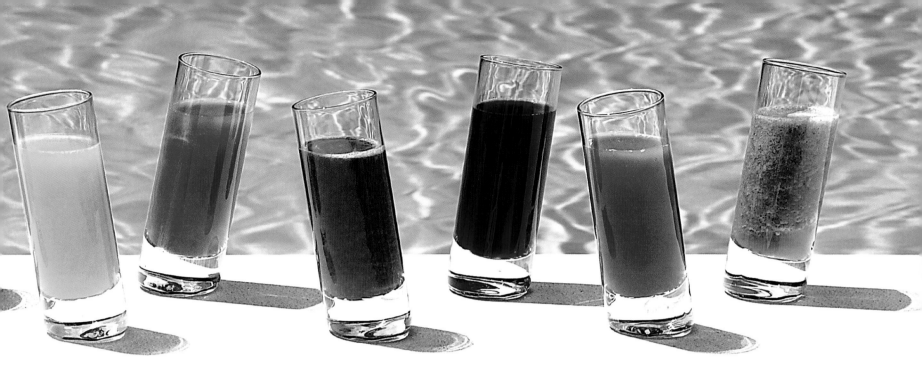

ANISE TEA

425 ml / ¾ pint / 2 cups of water, boiling
1 tsp dried anise leaves
1 tsp wild honey
Steep anise leaves in boiling water for about
5–6 minutes. Strain, sweeten with honey and
serve hot.

CALMING HERB TEA

1 tsp dried peppermint leaves
1 tsp dried lemon balm leaves
425 ml / ¾ pint / 2 cups boiling water
2 tsp wild honey
Add leaves to a warmed teapot and pour in
boiling water. Cover and steep for about 5
minutes. Strain and serve, sweeten with honey if
desired for a soothing herbal tea.

CAMOMILE HERB TEA

2 tbsp fresh camomile flowers
425 ml / ¾ pint / 2 cups boiling water
2 thin slices of green apple
2 tsp wild honey
Rinse the flowers with cool water. Warm teapot
with a little boiling water. Place apple slices in the
pot and mash them with a wooden spoon. Add
camomile flowers and pour in boiling water.
Cover and steep for 3–5 minutes. Strain and serve,
sweeten with honey if desired.

COOLING PEPPERMINT TEA

30 g / 1 oz peppermint
A few slices of lemon
Add peppermint to a teapot of boiling water. Top
with a few slices of lemon and let it steep covered
for about 10 minutes before serving hot.

FRESH GINGER TEA

5 cm / 2-inch piece of fresh ginger, peeled and
grated
1 L / 1¾ pints / 4 cups boiling water
Wild honey to taste
Place ginger in teapot and pour in boiling water.
Allow to steep for 5 minutes, and strain. Serve hot
and sweeten with honey and lemon if desired.

LAVENDER HERB TEA

1 tsp dried lavender flowers
1 tsp dried camomile flowers
1 tsp green tea leaves
1 L / 1¾ pints / 4 cups boiling water
2 tsp wild honey, to taste
Place herbs in a warmed teapot and pour in
boiling water. Cover and steep for 3–5 minutes.
Strain and serve, sweeten with honey if desired.

MINT AND LEMON ICED TEA

4 black teabags
700 ml / 1¼ pints / 3 cups boiling water
2 sprigs of fresh mint
Juice of 2 lemons
1.2 L / 2 pints / 5 cups cold water
1–2 tbsp wild honey, to taste
Fresh mint and sliced lemon for garnish
In a teapot, brew the black tea in boiling water
with the mint for 5 minutes. Remove teabags and
mint, and add honey and lemon juice, stirring until
dissolved. Stir in cold water. Serve over ice, garnish
with mint leaves and a slice of lemon.

PEPPERMINT-FENNEL TEA

225 g / 8 oz peppermint leaves
225 g / 8 oz lemon balm leaves
225 g / 8 oz fennel seeds
Mix herbs thoroughly, and store in an airtight
container. Use 1 tsp of herb mixture for each cup
of boiling water. Steep for 10 minutes and strain
the herbs before drinking. Herb mixture can keep
for a few weeks.

REFRESHING TEA

1 tbsp camomile leaves
1 tbsp damiana leaves
1 tbsp chopped lemongrass
1 tbsp mint leaves
¼ tbsp jasmine flowers
¼ tbsp orange peel, grated
425 ml / ¾ pint / 2 cups
Combine herbs with two cups of water. Simmer for
15 minutes, strain and serve hot.

SAGE-LEMON TEA

1 L / 1¾ pints / 4 cups boiling water
1 tbsp fresh sage leaves
2 tsp wild honey
2 tsp grated lemon zest
Juice from one lemon
Keep water at a simmer, and add sage, honey
lemon zest and juice. Steep for 30 minutes. Strain
herbs and serve hot or iced cold.

SPICED & HERBAL TEA

3 tsp grated ginger
1 tsp coriander seeds
A pinch of cinnamon powder
2 cardamom pods
A pinch of allspice
2 tsp dried camomile flowers
Combine all ingredients, except camomile, in a
small saucepan of water, bring to a boil and
simmer for 20 minutes. Remove from heat and
add camomile. Steep for another 10 minutes.
Strain herbs and serve hot.

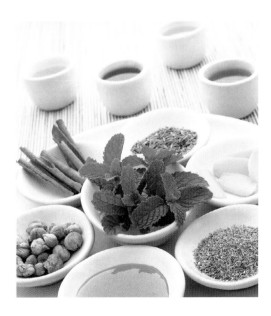

DRESSINGS

MUSTARD DRESSING

½ onion, finely chopped
½ green apple, finely chopped
2 slices ginger, finely chopped
100 ml / 3½ fl oz / ⅜ cup white wine or cider vinegar
4 tbsp shallot or tarragon vinegar
2 tbsp Dijon mustard
3 tbsp wholegrain mustard
200 ml / 7 fl oz / ⅞ cup grapeseed oil
100 ml / 3½ fl oz / ⅜ cup walnut or hazelnut oil (if unavailable replace with olive oil)
80 g / 2¾ oz crème fraîche
100 ml / 3½ fl oz / ⅜ cup basic stock (see recipe on this page)
Herbal salt substitute (see recipe on opposite page), to taste
Freshly ground black pepper, to taste
1–2 tbsp honey

Combine onion, apple and ginger with vinegars. Next add mustards and slowly pour in all the oils, stirring continuously. Mix thoroughly and add crème fraîche and stock. Season with honey.
To adapt recipe to a curry dressing, replace mustards with 1 tbsp madras curry powder and combine ingredients over a medium heat to release flavours. Dressings can be stored in an airtight container for a few weeks.

TOMATO DRESSING

6 tomatoes, cut into wedges
1 tbsp tarragon leaves
Handful of basil leaves
½ red onion, finely chopped
3 cloves garlic, finely chopped
200 ml / 7 fl oz / ⅞ cup tomato juice
100 ml / 3½ fl oz / ⅜ cup white wine vinegar
300 ml / ½ pint / 1¼ cups olive oil, chilled in the freezer
A pinch of herbal salt substitute (see recipe on opposite page)
A pinch of freshly ground black pepper
A pinch of sugar

In a frying-pan, heat tomato wedges in a little olive oil. Add tarragon, basil, onion and garlic and stir over a medium heat. Add tomato juice and vinegar and bring to a boil. Once boiled, remove from heat and set aside to cool. When ready, pour mixture into a glass bottle and pour in the ice-cold olive oil and shake vigorously. The coldness of the oil will allow the mixture to coagulate without the tomato mixture settling at the bottom of the bottle. Season with herbal salt, pepper and sugar.

ORANGE VINAIGRETTE

Zest of one orange
Juice and pulp of 120 g / 4¼ oz oranges
¼ leek, finely sliced
4 tbsp olive oil
1 tsp lemon juice
2 tbsp orange juice
Freshly ground black pepper, to taste

Blanch the orange zest twice, then mix all the ingredients in a bowl and refrigerate for 24 hours. Prepare in advance and store in the refrigerator.

HERB AND SPICE MIXES

BARBECUE SPICE MIX

2 tbsp paprika powder
1 tbsp chilli powder
1 tsp ground coriander
1 tsp ground cumin
1 tsp herbal salt substitute (see recipe on opposite page)
1 tsp sugar
½ tsp Madras curry powder
½ tsp dry mustard
½ tsp freshly ground black pepper
½ tsp cayenne pepper
½ tsp dried thyme leaves

Combine ingredients and store in a screw-top jar.

CAJUN SPICE MIX

110 g / 4 oz herbal salt substitute (see recipe on opposite page)
3 tbsp chilli powder
3 tbsp paprika
2 tbsp dried basil
2 tbsp ground coriander
2 tbsp dried oregano
2 tbsp coarsely ground black pepper
2 tbsp onion powder
1½ tbsp dried thyme
¾ tsp cayenne pepper
½ tsp white pepper
⅓ tsp ground cumin

Combine ingredients and store in a screw-top jar.

DRY CHERMOULAH SPICE MIX

60 g / 2¼ oz breadcrumbs
½ tsp paprika
1 tsp cayenne pepper
½ tsp cajun powder
1 tbsp curry powder
½ tsp herbal salt substitute (see recipe on opposite page)
3 cloves garlic, chopped
Freshly ground black pepper, to taste
1 tbsp olive oil

Toast all ingredients together in olive oil until golden brown. This should take about 2 minutes, be careful as they can burn quickly. Store in an airtight container for up to 1 week.

WET CHERMOULAH SPICE MIX

10 cloves garlic, chopped
5 shallots, chopped
½ large red chilli, chopped
1 tsp coriander powder
1 tsp paprika powder
Juice of 1 lemon
Herbal salt substitute (see recipe on opposite page), to taste
Freshly ground black pepper, to taste
100 ml / 3½ oz / ⅜ cup olive oil

Chop garlic, shallots and large red chilli. Heat chopped ingredients in a little olive oil and simmer over a medium heat. Add coriander and paprika powder and allow to dissolve. Top with lemon juice and season. Add oil and mix well. Remove from heat and allow to cool. Marinade is then ready to use. Store in an airtight container in the refrigerator for up to 3 days.

FIVE SPICE POWDER

2 tbsp black peppercorns
2 tsp fennel seeds
3 pieces of star anise
2–3 cinnamon sticks, broken into small pieces
6 cloves

Using a pestle and mortar, grind all ingredients together. Store in a screw-top jar.

HERBAL SALT SUBSTITUTE

1 tbsp ground cayenne pepper
1 tbsp garlic powder
1 tbsp onion powder
1 tsp dried basil
1 tsp ground dried grated lemon peel
1 tsp ground mace
1 tsp dried marjoram
1 tsp dried oregano
1 tsp dried parsley flakes
1 tsp freshly ground black pepper
1 tsp dried sage
1 tsp dried savoury
1 tsp dried thyme

Mix ingredients together and keep in a salt cellar.

HERBS DE PROVENCE

3 tbsp dried marjoram
3 tbsp dried savoury
3 tbsp dried thyme
1 tsp dried basil
1 tsp dried rosemary
½ tsp fennel seeds
½ tsp dried sage

Combine ingredients and store in a screw-top jar.

MEXICAN SPICE MIX

3 tbsp chilli powder
1½ tbsp paprika
1 tbsp ground cumin
2 tsp dried oregano leaves
1 tsp ground dried red capsicum (fresh if possible)
1 tsp garlic powder
1 tsp herbal salt substitute (see recipe on this page)

Combine ingredients and store in a screw-top jar.

MOROCCAN SPICE MIX

Zest of 1 orange
2 tsp crushed hot chillies
2 tsp ground coriander
2 tsp ground cumin
2 tsp ground ginger
1 tsp coarsely ground black pepper
½ tsp ground cinnamon
½ tsp wild honey
½ tsp herbal salt substitute (see recipe on this page)
½ tsp turmeric powder

Mix all ingredients thoroughly. Store in a screw-top jar and keep for up to 3 days.

SAUCES

CORIANDER YOGHURT SALSA

1 bunch coriander
150 g / 5½ oz low-fat yoghurt
4–5 small green chillies or 2 jalapeño chillies
4–5 cloves garlic
1 tsp salt substitute (see recipe on this page)
125 ml / 4 fl oz / ½ cup water

Cut coriander into short lengths. Blend all ingredients together until just uniform but still a little chunky. Store in an airtight container in the refrigerator.

NORI-GINGER MARINADE SAUCE

1½ tbsp roasted sesame oil
1 large clove garlic, minced or pressed
1 sheet nori
1 tbsp ginger seasoning
½ tsp Chinese five-spice powder
½ tsp sesame oil

Whisk all ingredients together until thoroughly mixed. Can be stored in an airtight container in the refrigerator for three days.

PESTO
100 g / 3½ oz Spinach, blanched
60 g / 2¼ oz pine nuts
35 g / 1¼ oz basil
100 ml / 3½ fl oz / ⅜ cup soy bean oil or olive oil
4 tbsp basil oil
1 clove garlic
12 drops Tabasco
5 drops Basilico
A pinch of salt substitute (see recipe on this page)
A pinch of freshly ground black pepper

Using a food processor, blend all ingredients until desired consistency. Store in an airtight container.

SALSA VERDE

1 clove garlic
Freshly ground black pepper
A pinch of salt substitute (see recipe on this page)
1 bunch coriander
1 spring onion, chopped
2 small anchovies
1 tsp Dijon mustard
1 tbsp capers
4 tbsp extra virgin olive oil

Chop garlic and crush it with a pinch of herbal salt. Pound all ingredients in a mortar with pestle, except the oil, until mixture resembles a raw paste. Whisk in the olive oil, you may need a little more, until the sauce has a thick consistency.

SPICED YOGHURT RELISH

1 red onion, sliced
1 cucumber, sliced
2 tomatoes, seeds removed and sliced
Freshly ground black pepper
1 tsp cumin seeds, toasted
1 bunch coriander, chopped
400 ml / 14 fl oz / 1⅔ cups low-fat yoghurt

Combine onion and cucumber in a sieve, sprinkle liberally with salt and set over a bowl for 10 minutes. Rinse thoroughly and pat dry. Mix all ingredients. Refrigerate until needed.

STOCKS

BASIC STOCK
100 g / 3½ oz leeks
100 g / 3½ oz garlic
3 shallots
100 ml / 3½ fl oz / ⅜ cup olive oil
1 clove
1 bay leaf
1L / 1¾ pint / 4 cups water
Freshly ground black pepper, to taste

Peel and clean the leeks, garlic and shallots. Put in a large saucepan with the olive oil, clove, bay leaf and water. Bring to a simmer and cook for about 25 minutes. Strain and adjust the seasoning with salt and pepper. Stock can be used with meats, fish and stews. Can be prepared in bulk and frozen.

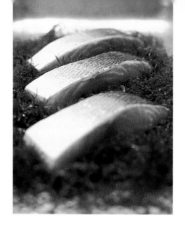

BUYING FISH

The eyes of fish should be fresh, bright and full; sunken, dull eyes are warning signs. Skin colour, too, should be bright and vivid; as a fish deteriorates, the colour dims. The fish should also have a covering of protective slime, which reduces as the fish gets older. Above all else, the smell should be an aroma of the sea. There should not be anything fishy about fish.

FARMED OR WILD?

Although there is nothing inherently wrong with farmed fish, how it is actually farmed is crucial. Habitat, diet and breeding all have an enormous influence on the final taste and flavour. You generally get what you pay for.

In a good supermarket the label on the fish should tell whether it is farmed or wild. Other tell-tale signs to look out for are uniformity of size, colour and shape.

FROZEN VERSUS FRESH

When fish is frozen it tends to lose some of its sweetness and flavour. If the freezing is done carefully this can be minimized. There is no such thing as quality cheap fish, so price is always a good guide. Those that are more expensive have been bought at the market, at a higher price and are therefore normally of superior quality.

SALTWATER AND FRESHWATER

Saltwater fish, such as brill, cod, Dover sole, grey mullet, red mullet, haddock, hake, halibut, herring, john dory, tuna, salmon* and sea bass, are from the sea.

Freshwater fish such as carp, pike, perch, river trout and eel come from rivers.

* Often called 'migrating fish', salmon are really a little of both. They travel huge distances throughout their lives. They are normally born in the river water and then swim out to the open sea before returning to the rivers to give birth.

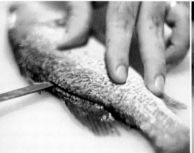 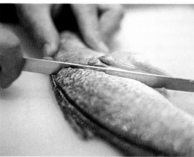 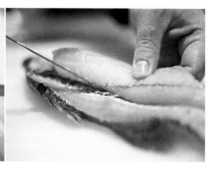

Preparing the fish before cooking will produce best results, as will buying ethically and avoiding those on the endangered list. OPPOSITE: Cooking lean meat that's covered with your favourite spices on a skewer is a healthy option.

BUYING MEAT AND POULTRY

While the demand for expensive cuts of meat continues to grow, the best chefs agree that more economical cuts can compete; they just require slower cooking. This technique will keep the meat tender and blend the flavours. Packed with protein, iron, zinc and essential vitamins, good quality meat should be healthy and vibrant in colour.

Once cooked, rest the meat and poultry to tenderize and give it a tasty, melt-in-the-mouth interior. About 15 minutes of rest time is recommended although larger pieces of meat require longer. Remove meat from the oven just before it is completely cooked, or when it has reached the desired final temperature, as it continues to cook while resting.

BEEF

Beef should be moist, but not too shiny, with a healthy, plump look and a rich red colour and fine grain. The distinct and generous marbling of creamy white or yellowish fat—depending on the breed of the animal, its age and diet—should run through the meat, especially in the thicker parts. Remove wrapping and refrigerate beef on a tray or plate covered loosely with foil. Vacuum-packed beef may change from a rich red to a

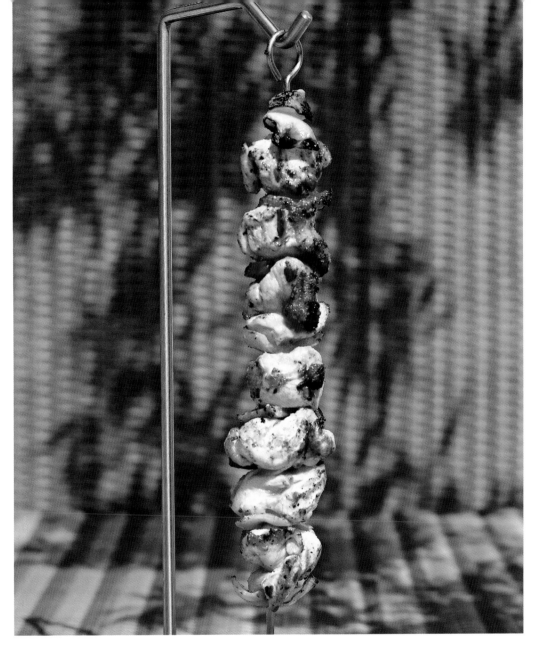

BUYING FRUIT AND VEGETABLES

When buying fruit and vegetables it is pertinent to remember that they are primarily composed of water, so if they look withered and dry, they probably are. Older produce tends to dehydrate quickly, so shop smartly to find the freshest, brightest and most flavourful produce. Buy in season when fruit and vegetables look and taste their best—they will be overflowing with nature's supernutrients.

While not always essential to pay over the odds for organic fruit and vegetables, if you are buying them it is worth ensuring that the produce is genuinely organic to justify the price tag attached. Organic farming does not necessarily mean that the product comes from sustainable sources.

Boiling and steaming are the classic and pure ways of cooking vegetables. Steaming perfectly complements the *Balancing Senses* recipes which call for fresh, colourful and nutrient-packed accompaniments. If boiling vegetables, ensure the water is in fact boiling with a pinch of sea salt or salt substitute added. Don't cover vegetables with the water—a small amount is all that is needed. Even with root vegetables like carrots and parsnips, water should only come to about three-quarters of the height of the vegetables.

A fast and healthy alternative is to use a high quality wok over a gas hob. Requiring just a splash of oil, this fast cooking technique ensures that the vegetables retain most of their supernutrient goodness while also giving you endless seasoning options.

Regardless of your chosen cooking method, do not overcook the vegetables; keep them crisp, colourful and crunchy with their nutritional benefits intact.

darker red or even grey once the pack is opened. This is normal and shows that no preservatives have been added. If a lot of juice or blood is released, the meat has most probably been frozen. Good quality chilled meat should not lose its juices.

VEAL When a calf is fed exclusively on its mother's milk, it gives a very pale pink meat, smelling of milk, with a satiny white fat. Slow roasted milk-fed veal rarely needs accompaniment other than sautéed or creamed spinach and pan-roasted potatoes. Before buying veal it is advisable to check where it comes from and choose the free-range option, which is far superior.

LAMB Some lamb can be quite high in fat and although the trend is a move away from fat, much of it melts in the cooking and can be left behind in the pan. Lamb should have a healthy pink hue, with an even coating of firm off-white fat. Lamb that is too lean is seldom good. Younger lamb has a milder aroma.

PORK Healthy pork should look hearty, moist and quite fatty with pale pink flesh that is finely grained with creamy-white fat. Free-range pork is tastier than the regular bred variety. For example, organic bacon releases much less liquid, so it is moister and far tastier. Leaner pork is obviously healthier, so eat fattier pork in moderation for its superior taste and quality.

CHICKEN The difference between free-range and battery chickens is a move from ordinary to excellent. Buy free-range chickens from a reputable supplier and don't be afraid to ask where the chicken is from and how it was reared. Healthy chickens should be plump and rounded with a pinky white colour and a non-offensive smell.

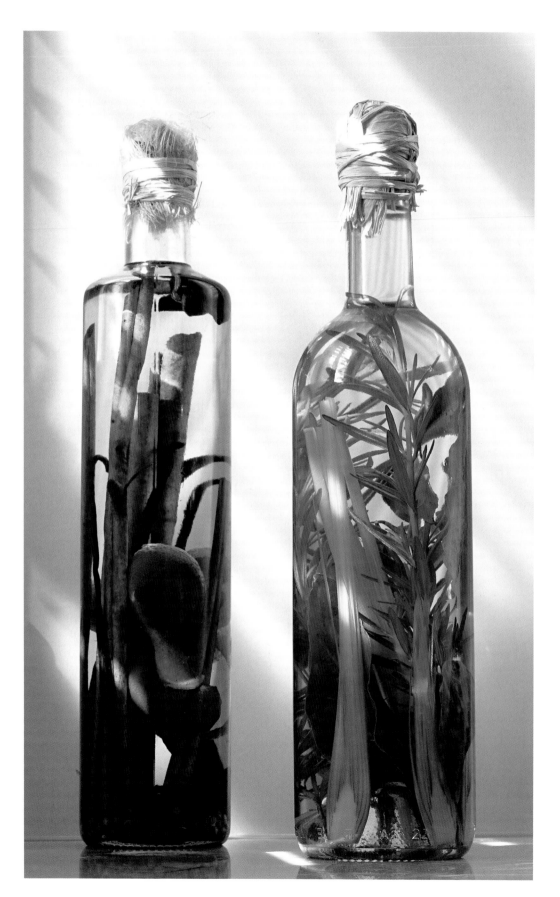

COOKING WITH OILS

While olive oil is the clear favourite even in the fussiest foodie's kitchen, there are plenty of other plants that produce good quality cooking oils. Nut and seed oils—such as walnut, hazelnut, groundnut oils and sesame and sunflower seed oils—offer a good alternative with very distinctive tastes.

When cooking with any oil, it is important to remember that when they are heated their characteristics change depending on their burning points. Sesame seed oil, for example, has a very low burning point and even a gentle heat can destroy the inherent qualities of the oil. The same is true of walnut and hazelnut oils. Others, like groundnut and sunflower oil, have higher burning points and tend therefore to be used widely in cooking—especially in Chinese cuisine where food is stir-fried at a relatively high temperature.

Many oils found in supermarkets today are intensely processed with little to no flavour remaining in the actual oil. To ensure you buy the best quality oil, look for smaller producers as their taste and content is often superior. If possible, taste the oil in the shop so you know exactly what you are buying.

As light, heat and damp are enemies of quality oils, turning them rancid, it is best to buy oil in smaller volumes and store away from light and heat in a cool and dry environment.

OLIVE OIL

Perhaps the most frequently used ingredient in cuisines worldwide, olive oil is available everywhere in varying degrees of quality. The colour of the oil varies from deep-cloudy green to light gold, while the taste can be pungent and peppery or fruity and light. When to use each is simply a matter of taste although, as most of the characteristics are lost on heating, using more expensive pungent oils for frying is a bit of a waste. It is much better to reserve these oils for dressings, or when the oil is consumed in its raw form.

Acidity is the culprit in bitter tasting oils; the higher the level of acid, the more fatty the oil will taste in the mouth. Low acidity gives a smooth and silky taste. Olive oil is generally graded based on this level of acidity.

While producers generally include a best-before date on bottles, oils have a maximum life of about 18 months and they begin to lose their fine qualities after about 12 months.

Choosing olive oil is a matter of personal taste but the following is a brief outline of the different types available to help make your choice easier.

EXTRA VIRGIN OLIVE OIL This oil is obtained from the first cold pressing of the olives; it is a virgin oil in that it is unprocessed. The oil must have a perfectly balanced aroma and flavour, colour and oleic acid content of 1 per cent or less.

FINE VIRGIN OLIVE OIL This oil must have a balanced aroma and taste and oleic acid content of less than 1.5 per cent.

SEMI-FINE OR VIRGIN OLIVE OIL Normally sold as 'virgin olive oil' with a maximum permitted oleic acid content of 3 per cent. Its aroma and taste must be good, as opposed to perfect.

PURE OR OLIVE OIL This is a combination of refined and virgin olive oil.

SINGLE ESTATE OILS Much like wines, these can vary from year to year but tend to have dominant characteristics that will soften through the year. Colour, too, will vary depending on the year, country of origin and colour of the olives used.

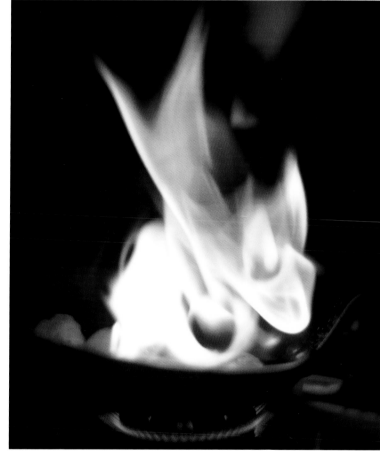

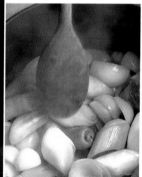

BLENDED OILS Can be either extra virgin or simply pure olive oil, these are the typical supermarket and own label brand oils designed to be consistent year on year. These are perfectly fine for using in most recipes in the home unless an extra-virgin oil is called for.

To spice-up the taste of a bland oil, simply add peeled garlic cloves, lemon zest, sprigs of herbs, chillies or toasted spices such as cumin or coriander. Allow the herbs to stand in the oil for one week. Strain and use in salad dressings and store in an airtight container.

Wok-frying is a quick and healthy way to cook vegetables as it keeps all the goodness inside.
OPPOSITE: Olive oil can be infused with herbs such as rosemary, basil, lemongrass, coriander and cumin, as well as spices such as cinnamon, for extra flavour.

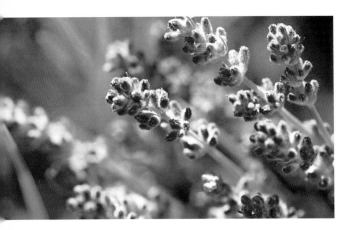

Oil from wild lavender helps relieve stress, anxiety and depression, it also helps to heal skin blemishes.
OPPOSITE (FROM LEFT): Sap from aloe vera leaves is used for its healing properties on the skin; While it's perfect with lamb, in aromatherapy, rosemary oil helps calm both body and mind.

HERBS

Fresh herbs are essential both for enhancing flavour and for the skin. While herbs are available in all corners of the globe, the quality is often debatable as many are harvested in vast greenhouses under artificial light and heat with the end result being tasteless and insipid. Use herbs at their freshest by growing them in the home. A window box, hanging basket that gets the sun, or simply a sunny window ledge is all that is required.

Generally herbs are better fresh as they lose their aroma and taste when dried. Oregano, thyme and bay, however, do dry well. When buying fresh herbs look for strong green, fresh and vibrant herbs that smell strongly if brushed.

DRYING HERBS

As most herbs are at their peak just before flowering, this is the best time to dry them. Choose a dry sunny day and cut herbs at the stem. Blanch and, to retain green colouring, tie whole stems very tightly in small bunches and hang upside down in paper bags in a dark room. This allows essential oils to flow from the stems to the leaves. When herbs are completely dry, place in airtight glass jars and store in a cool, dry place. For the first few days, examine the jars and check for moisture; herbs will mould quickly if not completely dry.

OVEN DRYING Place leaves or seeds on a flat sheet or shallow pan not more than one inch deep and dry at a very low heat (less than 80°C / 180°F for 2–4 hours.

FREEZING Although it is not ideal, herbs can be frozen for convenience. If freezing, wash thoroughly and blanch herbs in boiling water for 30 seconds. Chill quickly in iced water, dry them of any excess water, package and place in the freezer. Fresh dill, chives, and basil can be frozen without blanching.

COMMONLY USED HERBS

ANISE is an annual herb that grows up to ½ m / 2 ft high. The leaves and seeds have a warm, sweet liquorice taste and is best planted after all danger of frost has passed. The leaves are best used in salads and as a garnish, while the seeds can be used as a flavouring. The seed oil is used in cough medicine and lozenges.

BASIL is an annual herb, about 45 cm / 18 in tall, which grows easily from seeds. Pinch stems to promote bushy, compact growth and pick about 6 weeks after planting, or once they are large enough. Medicinally, basil is used to treat headaches, coughs, diarrhoea, constipation, warts, worms and kidney problems. Basil oil has antibacterial properties.

CHIVES are small, hardy perennials that belong to the onion family. They grow in clumps reaching about 25 cm / 10 in in height. Chives grow easily and demand little attention. The long leaves can be cut for use as they grow and impart a delicious, subtle, onion flavour.

CORIANDER is an annual plant that grows to ½ m / 2 ft high. The seeds are best sown in spring and the leaves can be picked when the plant has grown to at least 10 cm / 4 in tall. The leaves impart a delicate taste, while the perfumed seeds are used as a condiment. Once considered an aphrodisiac, it is used medicinally as a stimulant and carminative.

DILL is an annual that grows easily from seeds sown in early spring to ½–1 m / 2–3 ft high. Both the leaves and seeds are popular for flavouring meats, sauces, stews, pickles and vinegars. As a medicinal plant, dill is used as a diuretic, anti-spasmodic and a stimulant.

FENNEL is a perennial that grows to 1 m / 3–4 ft tall. The best stems for eating are the tender flower stalks just before they blossom. Fennel

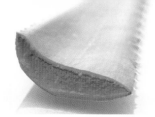

seeds are used in cheese spreads and vegetable dishes. The leaves have a liquorice flavour and the stems can be eaten like celery. The seeds are used as a diuretic, laxative, antispasmodic, expectorant, and to stimulate a mother's milk production.

GINGER is a rhizome. It's leafy plant extends about 1 m / 3 ft above ground and is best planted in spring in a lightly shaded area with rich, moist but well-drained soil. Soak the tubers overnight in warm water first then set them just under the soil's surface with the buds facing upwards. Ginger has a refreshing, lemon aroma and a warm, slightly sweet taste. It is ideal in a hot cleansing tea and adds richness and depth to cooking. Ginger is widely used in TCM to combat damp-related imbalances such as rheumatism, arthritis, muscular pain and fatigue. Ginger tea helps relieve colds, flu, stomach cramps and nausea.

LEMONGRASS is a perennial herb that grows in a warm and humid climate with leaves up to 1 m / 2 ft long. It grows well in sandy soils with adequate drainage. Fragrant and lemony, lemongrass is best used in teas, clear soups and is widely used to add flavour to fish, chicken and pork dishes in Thai and Indonesian cuisine. The oil is extracted for perfumes and cosmetics, such as soaps and creams. As a medicinal plant, lemongrass freshens the mind, it's traditionally considered a carminative and also makes an excellent insect repellent.

MARJORAM is one of the most fragrant herbs. It reaches a height of up to 30 cm / 1 ft and spreads. In colder climates, it is best treated as an annual or kept over winter as a pot plant. Marjoram is widely used to flavour fish, meats, salads, soups, eggs and

HOW ORGANIC IS ORGANIC?

Organic agriculture is defined as an ecological production management system that promotes and enhances biodiversity, biological cycles and soil biological activity. But the word is meaningless unless it is linked to a recognized scheme such as The Soil Association or British Organic Farmers and Growers in the UK, or the equivalent in other countries. Sadly, the term is sometimes abused for commercial advantage. While organic practices cannot ensure that products are completely free of residues, the methods used aim to minimize pollution from air, soil and water. However in many countries, measures to control organic production are not very efficient or may be unclear, which—coupled with insufficient knowledge—contributes to the food not being entirely organic.

What is generally meant by organic is in many ways a return to the past—something grown in a field, fed natural ingredients and harvested when nature dictated. However, in the case of many of the organically labelled fruits and vegetables on sale today, they are grown so far away that they lose much of their goodness by the time they get to your kitchen. If you choose to buy organic, then ensure your local retailer can justify the price tag by asking where the product was grown, when it was picked and is it really organic. Once you are satisfied with their response you will be more certain that what you are buying is really doing you and your family some good.

vegetables, and should be added towards the end of cooking. The oil is used to make perfume and is believed to warm the emotions and dispel agitation. It's also a folk remedy for asthma, indigestion, headache and toothache.

OREGANO is a hardy perennial with stems that can grow up to ½ m / 2 ft tall. It grows well even in poor soil and foliage can be stimulated

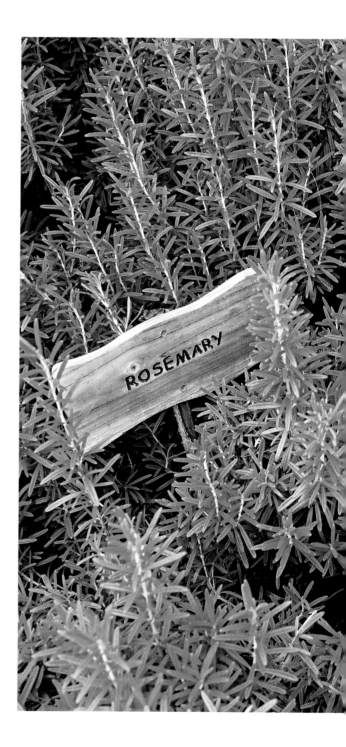

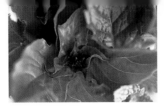

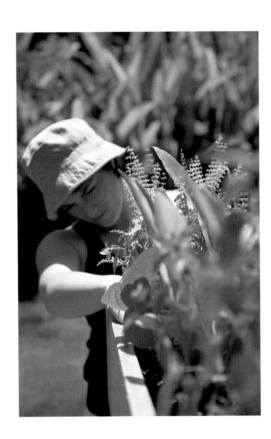

Outdoor herb gardens thrive in sunny and well-drained locations—a window box is ideal.
OPPOSITE: Sage, rosemary and thyme are hardier herbs that stand up to cooking.

AN INDOOR HERB GARDEN

Herbs can be grown in containers, window boxes, or hanging baskets in the home. Seeds should be sown in shallow boxes in late winter or very early spring in a light, well-drained soil mix that is not too rich. As a general rule, the finer the seed, the shallower it should be sown. When planting, mix two parts sterilized potting soil with one part coarse sand or perlite. For extra soil sweetness add 1 tsp of lime per pot and to ensure adequate drainage, add gravel at the bottom of each pot.

Lighting and watering are the most important consideration with herbs. Place them by a sunny window and, though they need water, do not drown them.

Annual herbs can spend their full life cycle in a pot indoors or on a window ledge. Hardy perennials thrive best outdoors during the warmer summer months; simply plunge the pot in soil up to its rim. Return indoors before the first frost to avoid plant damage. Fresh leaves can be picked as soon as the plant has enough foliage to maintain growth.

by simply cutting back the flowers. Oregano is the perfect partner for pizza and the leaves can be sprinkled over lamb or steak and added to Italian-style sauces. It is best to add towards the end of cooking.

PARSLEY is a biennial herb that grows easily with a characteristic flavour and smell that's great for garnishing or flavouring. Medicinally, parsley is an antispasmodic and diuretic, and helps relieve asthma, fever and jaundice.

MINT has several varieties but the most widely used are spearmint and peppermint. The leaves of the various mint varieties are the perfect partners for lamb, peas, tea and fruit drinks. Spearmint is used principally in mint sauce, while peppermint is more commonly used as a remedy for digestive upsets, indigestion and vomiting. Warming and stimulating, mint also helps ease the symptoms of colds and flu.

ROSEMARY is a hardy perennial, with a spicy, resinous fragrance. It grows best in well-drained, sunny locations in a lime-rich soil. Rosemary is great for flavouring meats, roast potatoes and dressings or as a garnish for roasts. Oil from the leaves is used medicinally to relax body and mind, calm nerves and soothe headaches.

SAGE is a woody perennial plant that grows ½–1 m / 2–3 ft tall and has a tendency to sprawl. Sage is best planted in direct sunlight and should be renewed every 3–4 years. Fresh and dried leaves of clary sage are used as flavouring agents in herbal teas and drinks as well as for stuffing, sausages and fish. The essential oil is extracted for perfume. Medicinally, sage is best known for its mucilaginous seeds that are used to clear sight and reduce inflammation of the eye area.

TARRAGON is a herbaceous perennial that grows to about ½ m / 2 ft in height. It will grow in full sun but thrives in semi-shade and needs protection during colder months. Tarragon leaves have a distinctive liquorice flavour and are used to season salads, marinades, sauces, stews, meat and fish. Medicinally, it is a diuretic and the roots are a folk remedy for toothache.

THYME is a wiry-stemmed perennial that reaches up to 25 cm / 10 inches in height. The stems are woody and leaves are small. Thyme is used for flavouring cheese, soups, stews, stuffing, meats, fish, dressing and sauces. Oil of thyme is used in perfume and medicinally as an antispasmodic and tonic to promote perspiration and dispel fever.

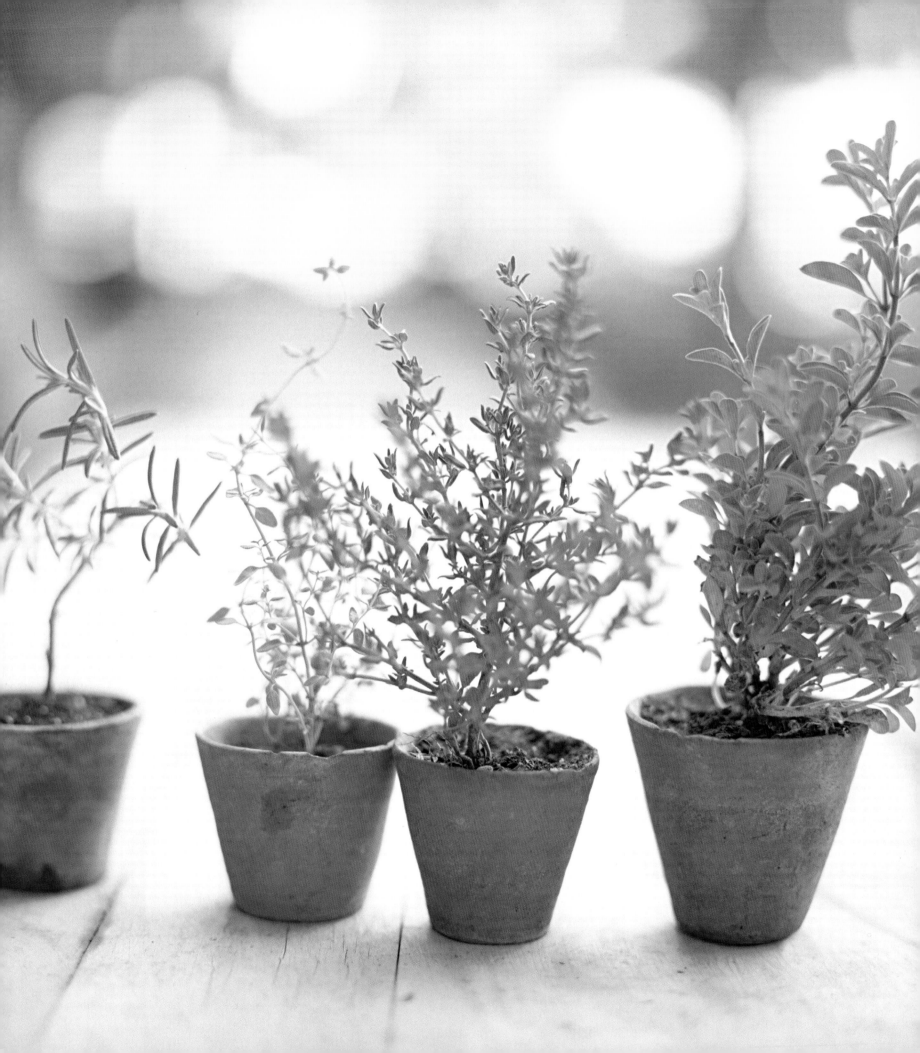

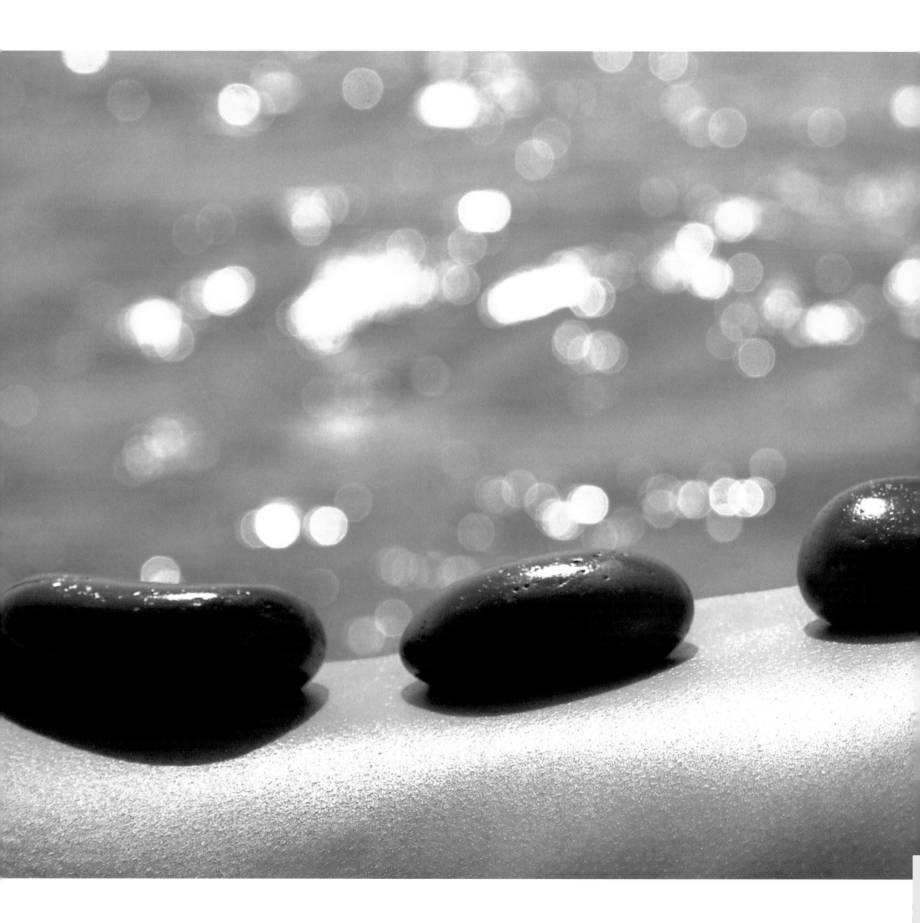

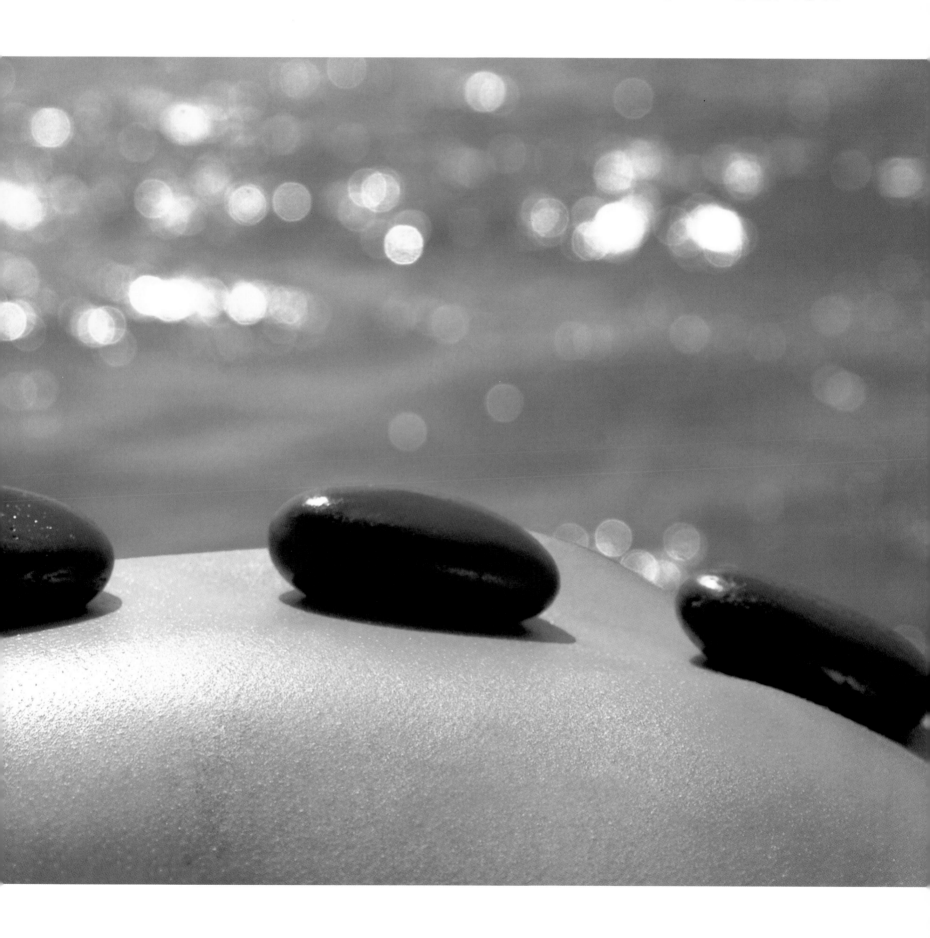

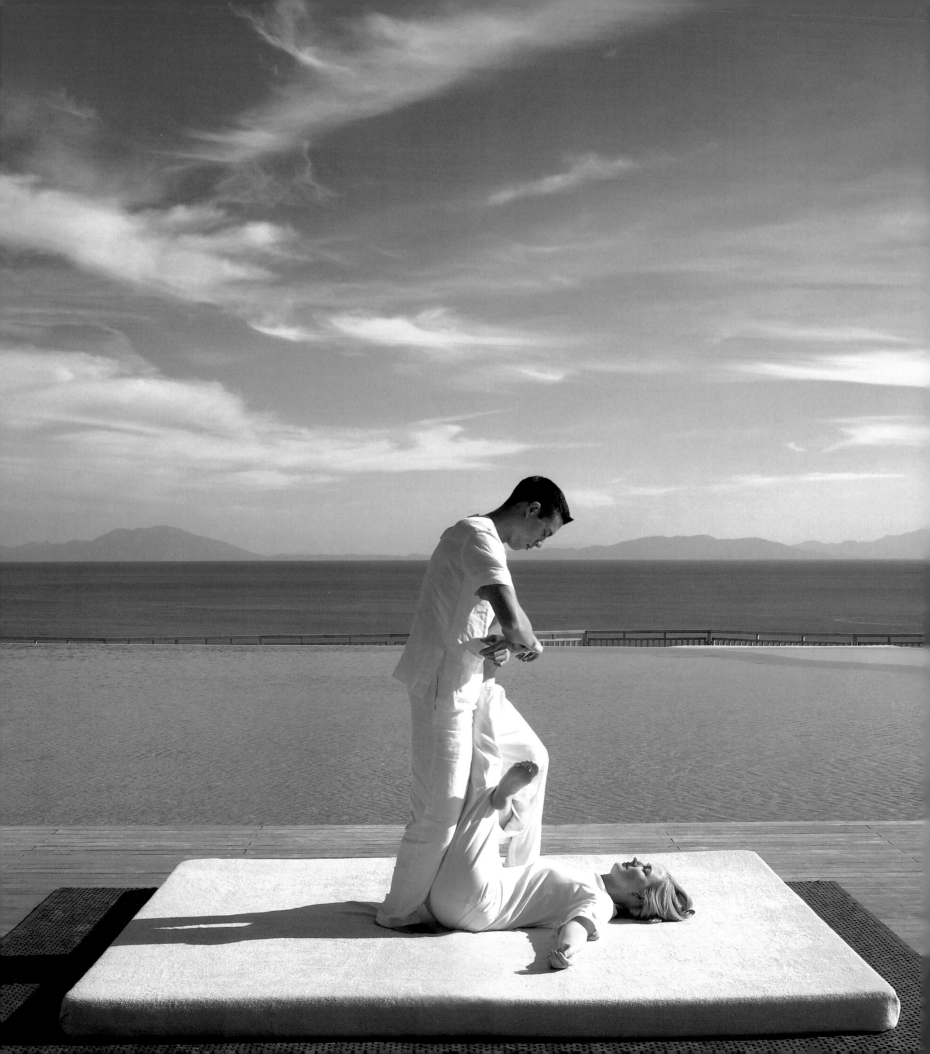

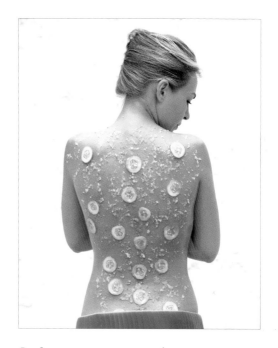

BEAUTY SENSE

When one tugs at a single thing in nature,
he finds it attached to the rest of the world.

-John Muir

When your skin and hair look good, you feel good. The good news is that working with *Balancing Senses* you can always look your best. The cycle of regularly losing and regaining weight experienced on most diets speeds up the ageing process, leaving the skin dull, tired and worn. *Beauty Sense* attacks the root causes of ageing, offering simple age-defying recipes and tips to help you look more alive, lose weight and keep it off while also maintaining radiantly healthy skin, hair and nails.

There is no denying that skin gets thinner with age, with total skin thickness decreasing by an estimated 6 per cent with every decade after the age of 30, and hair and nails become dry and brittle, especially when not adequately nourished and protected. Although lasers, Botox, fillers and a battery of other invasive intervention techniques have become essential ingredients in the skincare routine of many by helping to reverse the visible signs of ageing, it is only by working preventatively from within, eating foods that play vital roles in protecting, regenerating and rehydrating the skin that we truly keep the skin younger, firmer and more supple. *Beauty Sense*'s skin-specific and age-defying masks and scrubs complement these vital foods by maintaining a brilliantly healthy glow. The same applies to hair and nails, with an added super-nutrient boost from within, in addition to extra nourishment and care from the outside—with easy-to-prepare scalp treatments and soaks and scrubs for the hands and feet—you can face a bright and glowing future, without compromise.

Everyone appreciates the healing and soothing powers of massage. This tactile sense has been a fundamental part of life and the backbone of well-being for centuries. *Beauty Sense* uncovers the true benefits of the age-old power of touch, helping you decide what works best for you. Whether it be the uniquely ayurvedic style of rebalancing the *doshas*, Chinese acupressure, stretching Thai style, the long sensual strokes of Indonesian, or the dance-like movements of Hawaiian Lomi Lomi, the classic Swedish style or the subtle blend of therapeutic essentials oils skilfully stroking the body in an aromatherapy massage, all therapies are designed to clear blocked energy channels, release tension and harmonize your body, mind and spirit.

Before an omen arises,
It's easy to take preventive
measures.

-Lao Tzu, Tao Te Ching (c.1066–770BC)

The cooling and nourishing properties of cucumber, thanks to its high water content, mix with aloe vera gel to create a superb after-sun cooler.
OPPOSITE: Unlocking the knots with traditional Thai massage at the Six Senses Spa in Bodrum, Turkey.

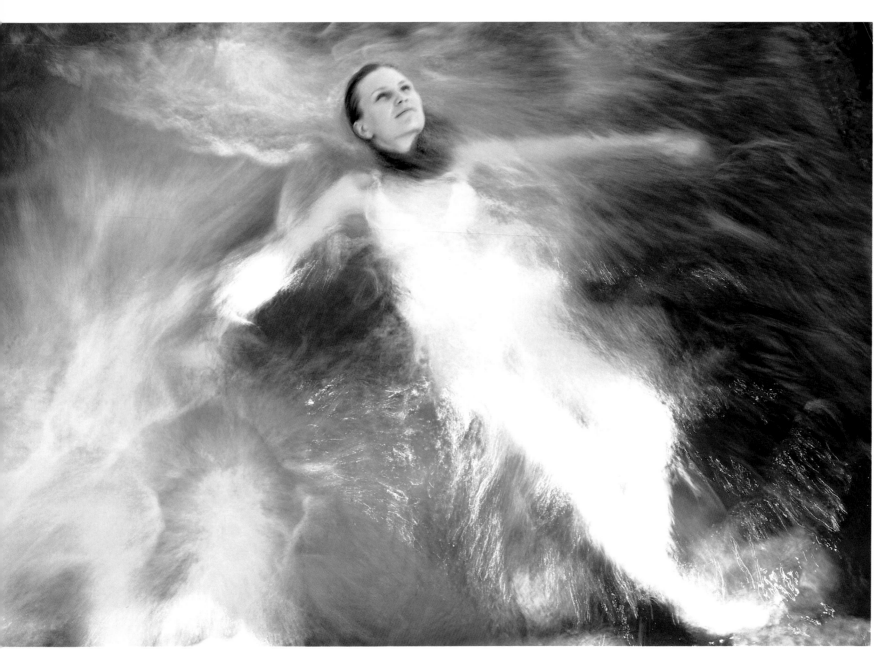

Make water a key element in your daily life, dehydration causes tired looking skin. OPPOSITE: Nourish the skin with an essential oil massage every week; A selection of freshly prepared face masks each packed with natural skin-vital goodness.

THE SKIN Achieving and maintaining a great complexion, while trying to hold back the effects of time and minimize blemishes, is possible as long as skin is adequately nourished from the inside out. Eating the *Balancing Senses* way not only helps you feel healthier and more vital, but results will be immediately apparent on the skin, too, as it quickly becomes clearer and smoother.

Collagen, which comprises 70–80 per cent of the skin's weight, and elastin are both essential for strong, elastic skin and the *Balancing Senses* supernutrient-packed menus are brimming with the necessary essentials for building and strengthening both.

The yo-yo cycle of diets that speeds up the ageing process combined with constant damage from the sun, pollution and daily life means skin is easily upset and prone to dryness, sagging and wrinkles. Stress alone dramatically ages the skin, giving it a dull, tired and lifeless look. Eating vital, fresh and seasonal foods protects, regenerates and rehydrates the skin, making it look and feel younger and glowing.

SKIN THROUGH THE DECADES

From the moment we are born we start to age but it is only in the twenties when the ageing effects become visible. Genetically programmed chronological ageing causes biochemical changes in the skin's collagen and elastin fibres. As each person's genetic programme is different, so too is the rate of skin ageing. This explains why some people age better than others. As skin becomes less elastic with the underlying fat padding starting to disappear, it becomes drier and starts to sag. Asian skin is stronger, tougher and less prone to wrinkles than Western skin, but it is not as supple.

THE TWENTIES Skin ageing in young adulthood is mostly limited to surface dehydration and dullness with some sun damage. Lifestyle factors rather than age are the main culprits here, as working and playing hard kick-starts the ageing process, as does pregnancy and the contraceptive pill.

THE THIRTIES Dehydration becomes more of a problem in the thirties. Also, the deeper layers of the skin start to thin out as collagen and elastin fibres begin to wear. The thirties signal the start of permanent lines, especially around the eyes and mouth.

THE FORTIES Skin changes become more dramatic in the forties with increased loss of elasticity, and gravity-induced sagging becomes more exaggerated. The overall result can be a tired-looking face hiding a vital personality. Asian skin is prone to age spots and pigmentation at this age.

THE FIFTIES AND BEYOND With the onset of menopause, skin becomes even more sensitive and dehydrated. Sunspots and pigmentation changes may be more noticeable as lines become more pronounced.

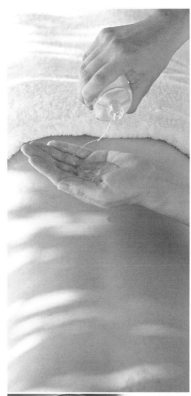

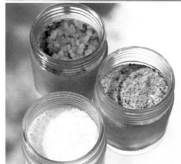

ENVIRONMENTAL HAZARDS

While you can't stop chronological ageing, you can do something to reduce skin damage caused by excessive sun exposure. Collagen provides the skin with a strong, firm texture and elastin maintains its resilience, but ultraviolet radiation from the sun produces free radicals that destroy this network thereby accelerating premature ageing. Always use sunscreen with an SPF of 15 or higher and ingredients like aluminium or zinc oxide that block both UVA and UVB rays. A higher factor would be needed on very hot days, especially in warmer climates. Stress, smoking, pollution and a diet of highly processed food are also culprits; together they disturb the body's natural balance resulting in tired and dull-looking skin. It is well known that smokers tend to have more wrinkles than non-smokers of the same age, complexion and sun exposure history.

PROTECT YOUR SKIN

There are various things you can do to avoid premature ageing of the skin:

- Always use a sunscreen with an SPF of 15 or higher and reapply frequently when you are in the sun.
- Always cleanse and tone the skin. Toning with an alcohol-free toner is essential to maintain the skin's natural acidity.
- Use moisturizer specific to your skin type, both morning and night.
- Wear large sunglasses and a hat with a brim to protect the hair, scalp and face when directly exposed to the sun.
- Make sure your daily moisturizer or foundation has an SPF of 15 or higher.
- Use nourishing and hydrating masks regularly, at least once a week (see skin food recipes on pages 94–6).

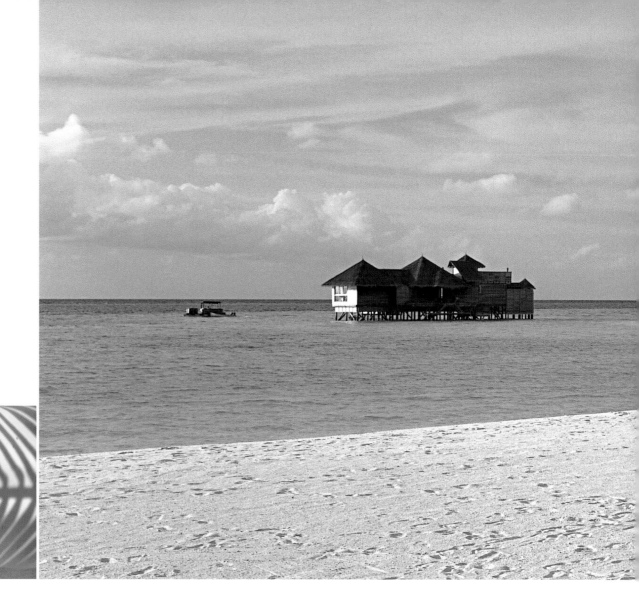

FEED YOUR SKIN While some people are fortunate to be born with great skin, most spend their lives trying to make it better. It has long been realized that for healthy skin, daily food and watering are essential, along with a nourishing skincare routine. One of the most common causes of dehydrated skin is lack of fluid. Water is essential, either on its own, with no ice, or as herbal tea or juices. There are also some nutrients to help you achieve glowing skin.

OILY FISH Salmon, trout and tuna are packed with omega-3 fatty acids which strengthen blood and keep skin cells watertight.

FRUIT AND VEGETABLES Eat plenty of apples, figs, berry fruits, apricots, avocados, bean sprouts, broccoli and other dark green vegetables, carrots, celery, chickpeas, ginger, green beans, plums, seaweed, spinach, sweet potatoes and squash.

GRAINS, NUTS AND SEEDS Eat plenty of brown rice, millet, sunflower seeds, whole grains, oats and walnuts.

LIVE YOGHURT The friendly bacteria in live yoghurt help maintain the body's natural acid mantle and combat the free radicals that are responsible for skin ageing.

SOYA In all its guises, soya is an excellent source of protein as well as being packed with phytoestrogens that help repair collagen and elastin and slow the rate of skin thinning.

OILS Safflower, flaxseed and wheatgerm oils are rich in EFAs, which help to maintain firm skin.

BRAZIL NUTS A few Brazil nuts a day, in cereal or as a snack, provide all the selenium the body needs. This is essential for making glutathione, an enzyme that zaps free radicals. Other selenium sources are tuna, shrimps, sunflower seeds, walnuts and cashew nuts.

FERULIC ACID Plants make this ferulic acid to protect them from the sun's damaging UV rays. It's said to have the same beneficial effects on human skin and is found in wholegrain cereals, berry fruits, apples, avocados and plums (see page 32).

OTHER SKINCARE ESSENTIALS

- Exercise maintains a healthy flow of blood and energy to the skin.
- Sleep is when the cellular repair of the skin is at its most active.
- Rest and relaxation help maintain an internal balance and stress-free skin.
- Essential oils help to maintain a healthy glow, use oils for your skin type (see page 111).

SOME ADDED NOURISHMENT In addition to your nightly cleanse, tone and moisturize, massage your face with a pure essential oil for your skin type. As it penetrates the inner cells, the oil stimulates circulation, helping to delay the onset of fine lines.

To create your own face oil add 25 drops of your oil to 25 ml / 1 fl oz almond-based oil; use sesame oil for dry skin. Dab a few drops in your hand, add a sprinkle of water and apply to moist skin. For the body, add 10 drops of oil to a base oil and apply to moistened skin.

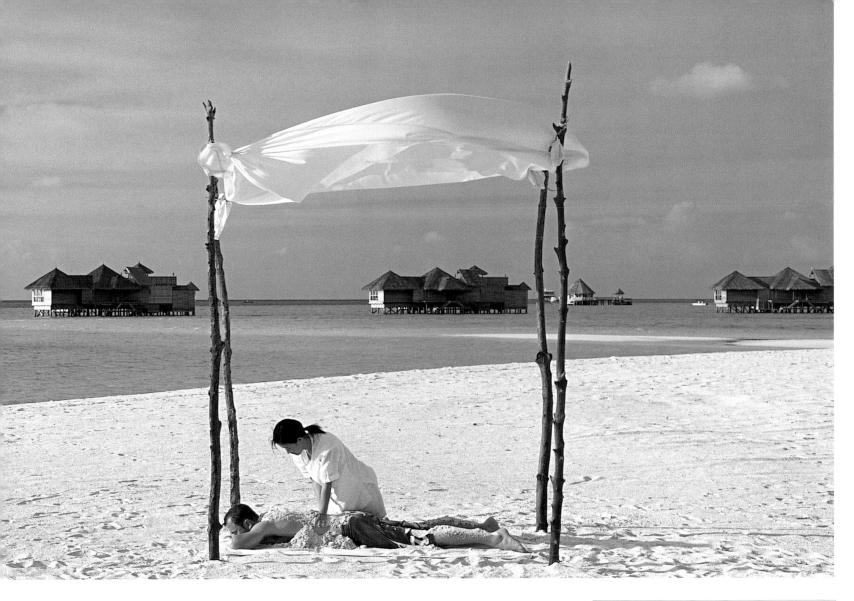

BE SHOPPING SAVVY: SKIN

The demand for natural and organic skincare has escalated in recent years as anxieties about preservatives, chemicals and environmental pollutants continue to manifest. Some beauty experts believe that with the continuing refinement in the extraction of properties from natural ingredients, the results and benefits of natural and organic skincare may soon overtake those of medically-based ingredients.

As each of us is an individual, requirements will differ and when choosing skincare products, the most pertinent advice is to let your skin decide. If it feels dry or rough then it probably is, and you will need to use a richer product and possibly apply more of it. Adjust your routine as the seasons demand, using added sun protection during hotter months and moisturizing more during very dry periods.

Most experts agree that the advent of the early thirties is the best time to switch to specific anti-ageing skincare products. Until then,

protect the skin against sun and environmental damage by moisturizing daily with an SPF 15, especially in sunnier climates. Always remember your large sunglasses and a wide brimmed hat when you are in the sun. It is far easier to prevent wrinkles than it is to erase them.

Be sure to scan labels before purchasing a new product. Try to avoid products containing petrochemicals, lauryl and laureth sulphates, propylene glycol, polyethylene glycols (PEGs), triethanolamine (TEA), diethanolamine (DEA), parabens, petrolatum and synthetic additives—all of which have health-related question marks surrounding them.

Products should be kept in a cool, dark place, away from direct heat and light. Once purchased, a product will normally have a shelf-life of up to 1 year—slightly less for active botanical and organic products or those designed for sensitive skins as these generally have fewer preservatives—after which the product will lose some therapeutic benefit.

FACIAL REFLEX ZONES

In Chinese medicine, imbalances in the body organs are evident in the face through the meridians represented in facial zones. For example, for women, a presenting symptom of hormonal imbalance is an eruption on the chin—the reflex zone for the kidneys, which are partly responsible for producing oestrogen.

- Forehead: Intestine
- Right cheek: Liver
- Left cheek: Lung
- Nose: Heart
- Mouth and Lips: Spleen
- Chin: Kidney

A full body massage set in the peaceful sanctuary of Soneva Gili in the Maldives. Making excellent use of natural resources, the fine-grain white sand is used for the highly effective body scrub treatments.

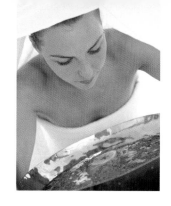

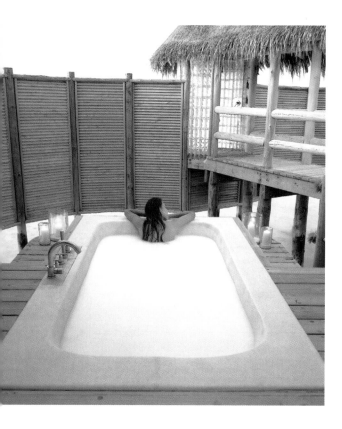

FROM TOP: A facial steam with lemon and flowers refreshes the skin; An aromatherapy bath at Soneva Gili.
OPPOSITE: The traditional hammam was a place of social gathering. While still a meeting place, the modern experience is a ritual with facial treatments, massage or other therapies.

SKIN DETOX As the body's largest organ, the skin is often the first to register toxic overload and a dull, pale and blemished appearance. While the 10-Day detox (see page 41) cleans the body from the inside, real skin cleaning means getting rid of the dead cells and allowing skin to renew and breathe more efficiently. Although skin cells are constantly being shed every day, body brushing stimulates circulation leaving the skin softer, cleaner and healthier. Also, facial steaming—using 2 cups of boiling water, the juice of half a lemon and a handful of fresh rose petals—is a wonderfully deep cleanser that leaves the skin refreshed and invigorated. Ginger- and pepper-rich foods help to eliminate toxins through perspiration, while ginger and cardamom tea is the perfect complement to a skin detox.

CARDAMOM AND GINGER TEA Mix cardamom and shavings of ginger in a cup with boiling water. Steep for 4–5 minutes. Add honey to taste and drink 2–3 cups per day.

PREPARING AND APPLYING MASKS Use organic fruits whenever possible, mashed and drained of juices. Ideally, masks should be applied onto freshly cleansed, slightly damp skin, avoiding contact with the eyes. Make the most of this time by lying back, placing a pillow under your knees for support and listening to your favourite music. Remove masks with lukewarm water or make your own herbal infusion of camomile and lime leaves that's been cooled to body temperature and strained. A gentle splashing of the infusion onto the skin will remove the mask. Allow the face to dry naturally; if you use a towel to dry your face, ensure it is soft and gently pat the skin to prevent it from stretching the skin.

OILY SKIN Although fortunate to reduce the appearance of fine lines and wrinkles, those with an oily complexion are more prone to acne, enlarged pores and blemishes. The key to effective skincare is to regulate oil production and calm the skin.

OILY SKIN: DO Cleanse the face twice a day with an alcohol-free liquid or gel cleanser. Use a moisturizer containing oil-controlling ingredients and an oil-free sunscreen with an SPF of 15 every day. Essential oils for oily skin include lavender, lemon, basil, juniper, geranium and ylang-ylang.

OILY SKIN: DON'T Make sure you don't overscrub the skin or use harsh cleansers that completely erase all surface oil. Oil is actually a protective barrier. Avoid cleansing the face more than twice a day. Don't use powder to soak in oil, it gives the skin a chalky appearance and can promote further oil secretion.

LEMON AND GRAPE MASK In the following recipe, the citrus of the lemon acts as a toner and antiseptic, the grapes moisturize and nourish and the egg white works on tightening the skin. This recipe can also be used on the oily areas of combination skin.
1 egg white, free-range if available
1 handful of seedless white grapes or 1 large ripe pear
Juice of ½ a lemon
1 tsp bran
Beat the egg white until it forms peaks. Peel and mash the grapes or pear and drain all the juices. Mix the egg white with lemon juice, bran and mashed fruits until the mixture becomes fluffy. Gently massage the mask onto cleansed skin, paying particular attention to the oily areas. Leave on the skin for 15 minutes before rinsing with warm water.

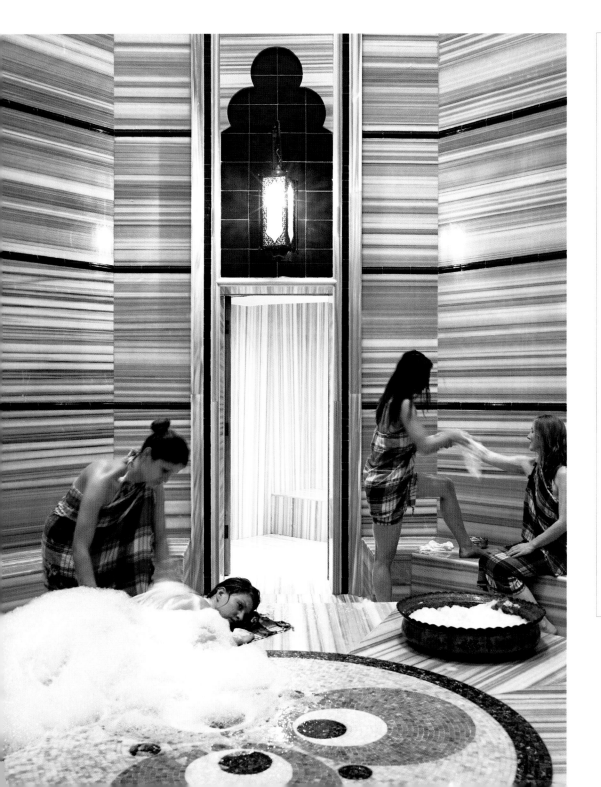

BATHING

From Rome to Egypt, from Indonesia to the Philippines and Japan, long languorous soaks are legendary. Cleopatra bathed in milk and honey. In ancient Indonesia, Javanese princesses regularly indulged in mandi susu, milk baths, to maintain soft smooth skin. Still now in Japan the onsen, (hot tub) is used exclusively for soaking—the body is scrubbed clean before getting into the bath—and a long soak at the end of the day has long been used to stimulate circulation, relieve stress and leave the body refreshingly clean. Around the world, bathing is still as popular as ever, both in spas and in the home, with specific essential oils, herbs or exotic flowers added to soothe and calm the body and mind.

HAMMAM

The hammam is the Turkish equivalent of the steam bath and flourished around the time of prophet Muhammad in 600AD. Being a place of social gathering and ritual cleansing, hammams were normally found close to the mosque or the souk, (Turkish marketplace). With the recent resurgence of bathing rituals, hammams are emerging in far-flung spas from Turkey and Egypt to London and Hong Kong. The modern hammam is normally part of a ritual that combines bathing with massage, stone therapy and even facials. The ritual takes place in a fully tiled majestic chamber, often complete with classically styled skylight columns, where the walls, floor and lounge benches are steam-heated. At the same time, aromatherapy essences such as eucalyptus disperse automatically into the moist atmosphere to deeply cleanse and revive the body.

ACNE Acne, an oily skin problem, is caused by blockages in the glands that produce the skin's protective oil or sebum. It can also arise, or be exacerbated by, hormonal imbalance—particularly during adolescence—and poor dietary habits, as well as emotional upset, radical climate changes and poor hygiene.

While much controversy exists over the role of diet in the development and control of acne, it is safe to say that by living and eating the *Balancing Senses* way, you are doing the very best you can to control acne through diet. Specific foods that might help control symptoms include sweet potatoes, carrots, mangoes and peaches. All are rich in beta-carotene which, when converted into vitamin A, may help reduce symptoms. Zinc-rich foods such as oysters, pine nuts, sesame seeds and cashew nuts help wound healing. Tea tree oil has potent antibacterial properties and helps control infection and inflammation—apply it sparingly to the affected area twice a day.

DRY SKIN Skin that suffers with dryness produces less oil and is therefore more prone to fine lines. It's common for women who are experiencing the menopause, and those prone to hormonal irregularities, to suffer with extremely dry skin, hair and eyes and an overall dehydrated countenance.

Drinking plenty of fluids—especially water—is important, as is the kind of food you eat. Oily fish, avocado, papaya, ginseng, sunflower and sesame seeds, soya-based foods, flaxseeds, ginger and jelly textured foods such as royal jelly and gelatine, should be part of an everyday diet. All of these foods will help firm and strengthen the skin, leaving it moisturized, hydrated and positively glowing.

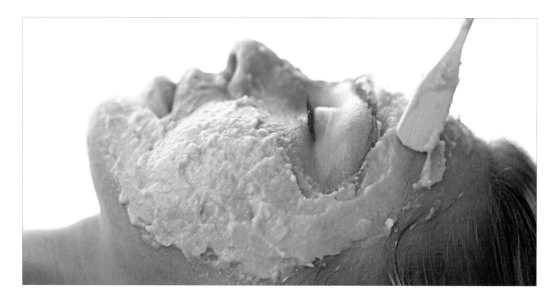

DRY SKIN: DO Use a mild, soap-free liquid or cream cleanser to wash the face once a day. In the morning just splash the face with warm water. Select moisturizers that delay moisture loss, like those containing hyaluronic acid or glycerine. Always apply your moisturizer when the face is still damp to lock in the moisture. Always use a sunscreen with an SPF of 15 or greater and reapply frequently, especially when in the sun. Oil-based foundations are best for softening fine lines. Essential oils for dry skin include sandalwood, geranium, rose, jasmine and camomile and lavender. For added nourishment, add 2 drops of your essential oil to your daily moisturizer.
DRY SKIN: DON'T Never wash your face with harsh soaps, and avoid grainy cleansers.
AVOCADO MASK This mask is packed with protein, vitamins, lecithin and essential fatty acids. If extra moisture is needed, add a little coconut oil. This recipe can also be used to nourish dry hands. Just make double the amount and use on face and hands simultaneously.

½ avocado, peeled and pitted
1 tbsp natural or plain yoghurt
1 tbsp coconut oil, optional
Mash the avocado with yoghurt and mix well. If preferred, combine them in a blender. Apply to cleansed skin and leave for 5–10 minutes before rinsing with warm water.

COMBINATION AND SENSITIVE SKIN Skin with an oily T-zone across the forehead and nose combined with a dry to normal complexion will benefit from eating general skin foods and drinking lots of water.
COMBINATION SKIN: DO Choose cleansers specifically formulated for combination skin; they are gentler on dry areas and tougher on oily patches. Use moisturizers formulated for sensitive skin, and foundations should be water-based or oil-free. Always use sunscreen with an SPF of 15 or greater, and reapply frequently. Essential oils suitable for combination skin include sandalwood, ylang ylang, mint, coriander, camphor and cumin.

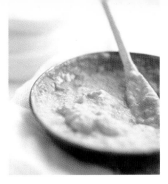

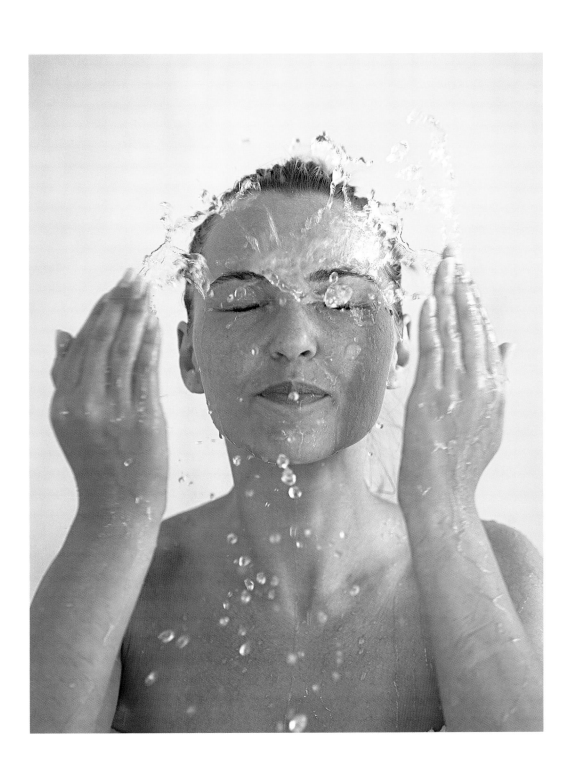

BUYING FOR YOUR SKIN TYPE

Always test a new product on an area of your skin that is generally hidden before applying it to the face. As the skin on the elbow is similar to the skin on your face, it is ideal for testing. Ingredients to look for:

DRY SKIN

Look for sulphate-free and soap-free cleansers with hydrating plant extracts such as aloe, rose and camomile essential oils. Choose heavier weighted moisturizers that contain oils such as lavender, geranium, rose and camomile.

OILY SKIN

Citrus fruits like lime and lemon are toning and antiseptic. Essential oils of rosemary, camomile, ylang-ylang and lavender help to reduce and balance the sebum production. A lightweight face serum is the best skin balancer.

COMBINATION AND SENSITIVE SKIN

Camomile and melissa essential oils and green tea products are very beneficial for both combination and sensitive skin. Overall, simple is best for sensitive skin types, meaning fewer ingredients and products on the skin. Always look for moisturizers with skin-calming ingredients such as vitamins A, C, and E and essential oils of patchouli, neroli, lavender and rosewood, all of which reduce sensitivity and stimulate cell renewal.

FROM TOP: Some freshly prepared anti-ageing face and eye mask; A healthy splash of water, essential to life and vitality.
OPPOSITE: A fresh avocado mask makes the perfect moisturizer for dry skin.

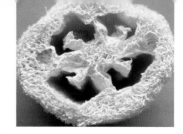

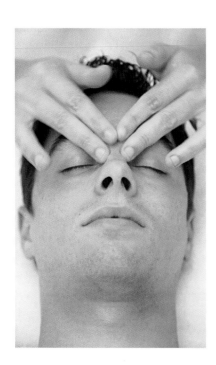

FROM TOP: Daily exfoliating with a loofah will keep the body free of dead skin cells; Massaging the reflex zones around the eyes will help ease stress, tension and headaches.
OPPOSITE: The nourishing nut body scrub, packed with essential oils, is the perfect nourishment for dry skin.

COMBINATION SKIN: DON'T Never use different cleansers and moisturizers for different parts of the face.

STRAWBERRY MINT MASK Strawberries—packed with natural antioxidants—soften the skin and assist in balancing oil production in normal or combination skins. Use this recipe once a week to help combination skin.

6 large ripe strawberries
1 handful of spearmint leaves
1 tsp wheatgerm oil
1 tsp orange juice

Blend the strawberries and spearmint leaves. Add the wheatgerm oil and orange juice. Spread the mixture evenly onto cleansed face and leave for 5–10 minutes before rinsing away with warm water.

THE EYES The eyes may indeed be the windows to the soul but in Chinese medicine a skilled physician can determine much about overall physical health by simply looking at the colour and life of the eyes. The delicate area around the eye is most prone to lines and wrinkles and everything from diet to stress; sleep and sun damage will determine how pronounced these lines are.

Pollution-induced, dry and blurry eyes not only make you look unattractive; they can be quite distressing, making balanced eating even more vital to scavenge those toxins. While the *Balancing Senses* menus will keep eyes nourished, apricots, avocados, berry fruits, oily fish, capsicums, spinach and other greens, wheatgerm and nuts help maintain moist, clear and bright eyes. Vitamin E in wheatgerm and carotenoid-rich foods such as carrots, mangoes and sweet potatoes helps protect the eyes from sun damage and pollution.

BE SHOPPING SAVVY: EYES Even more important when choosing eye care, you should scan ingredient labels before buying and steer clear of the ingredients listed on page 91. Irrespective of the product, a small amount should be massaged around the orbital bone around the eye zone, avoiding the immediate eye area itself. Too much or too rich a product can lead to puffiness and sensitivity.

ANTI-AGEING FACE AND EYE MASK
1 small banana
1 tbsp organic honey
1 tbsp oat flour
1 tbsp mineral water
2 tbsp natural yoghurt

Mash the banana and add the yoghurt, honey and oat flour. Stir in the water. For a thicker consistency, add more yoghurt or flour. Gently massage the mask onto the entire face and close to the eyes, yet avoiding their immediate surrounds. Leave for 15 minutes and rinse off.

THE BODY Just as the face is fed and nurtured daily, so too should the skin on the body as it is prone to dryness, lines and ageing almost as much as the face.

BE SHOPPING SAVVY: BODY Sodium lauryl sulphate and sodium laureth sulphate are harsh detergents that are commonly found in body washes and bubble baths, for both adults and children. They strip and irritate the skin, leaving it tight and itchy. For smooth and supple skin, scan labels and steer clear of the ingredients listed on page 91. A nourishing and aromatic option is a skin-specific essential oil-based bath oil packed with natural active ingredients that replenishes the skin as you bathe.

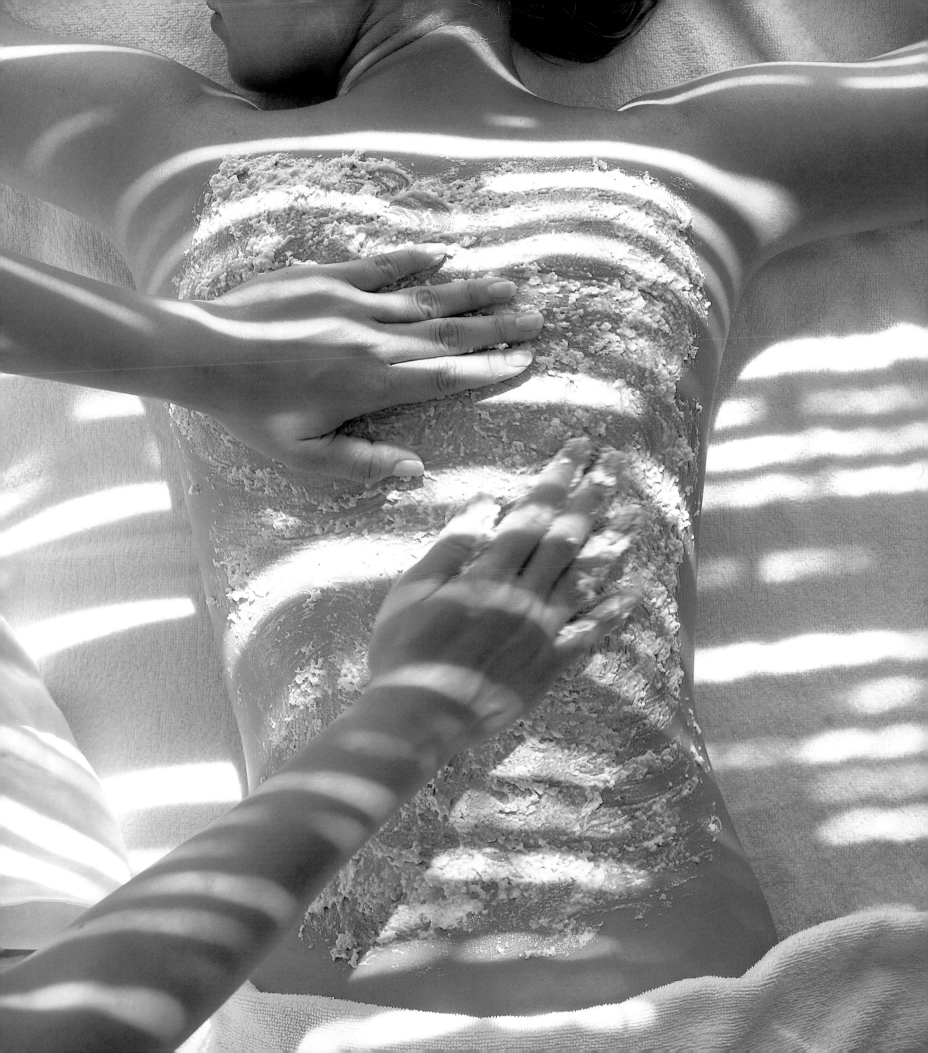

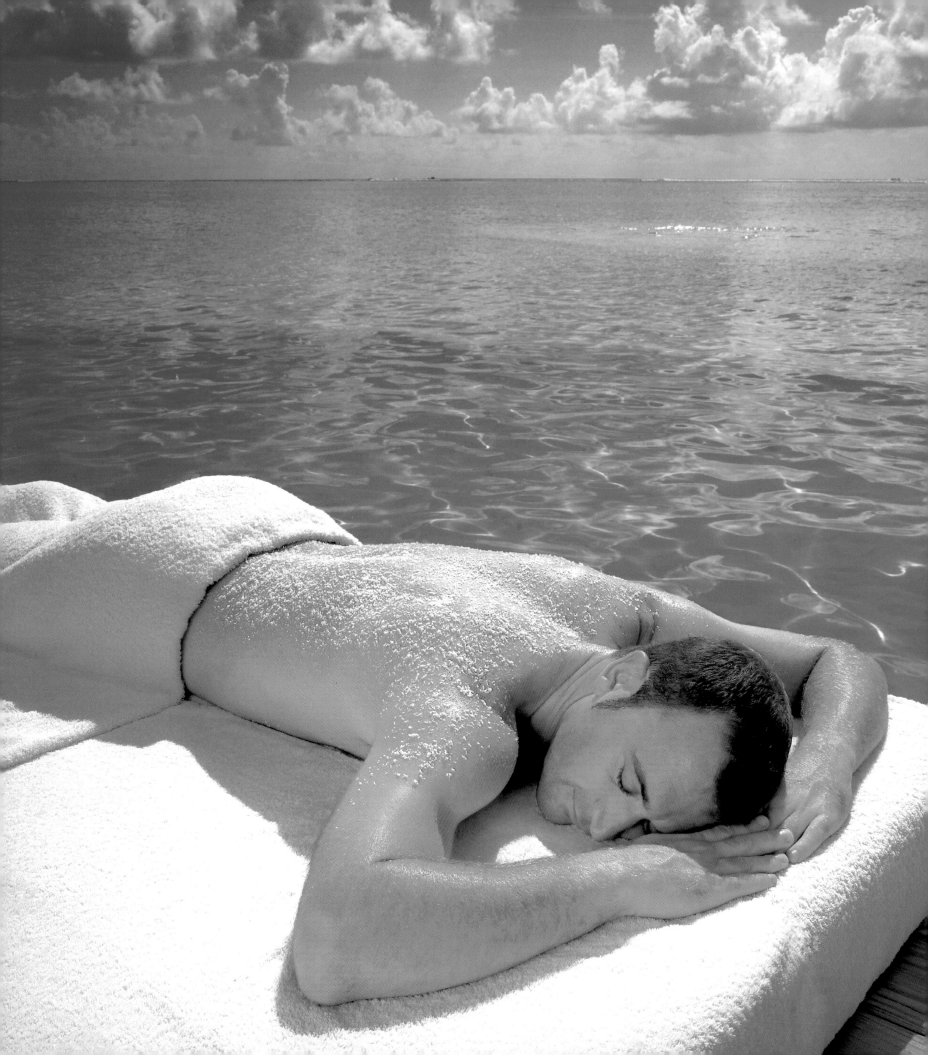

NOURISHING NUT BODY SCRUB

This recipe is suitable for all skin types, especially dry skin, due to the moisturizing effects of the nut oils

100 g / 3½ oz ground nuts such as almonds, walnuts or linseeds

50 g / 1½ oz flour

50 g / 1½ oz oatmeal

1 tbsp water, add more if required to attain the desired consistency

Combine all dry ingredients in a blender until a coarse mixture is achieved. Pour into a screw top jar. The scrub can be kept in a freezer. When you want to use it, remove 1 tbsp from the jar, add water and mix to make a paste. Rub in a gentle circular motion over the body to deeply exfoliate. Leave on the skin for about 5 minutes and rinse under a warm shower.

SKIN-SOFTENING SUGAR SCRUB

This is suitable for most skin types and will exfoliate, soothe and soften the skin.

250 g / 9 oz natural cane sugar

200 ml / 7 fl oz avocado oil, or vegetable glycerine

2 tsp aloe vera gel

3 drops lavender essential oil

2 drops orange essential oil

Combine all ingredients in a large bowl. Using your hand, scoop up some of the mixture and rub in a gentle circular motion over the body to exfoliate dead skin cells, making the complexion smoother. Leave on the skin for 5 minutes and rinse off under a warm shower.

SENSITIVE SKIN BODY SCRUB

This scrub is suitable for sensitive skin as it uses soft grains, which reduce the risk of a negative reaction. Those with normal skin can use it as well—it is ideal if you wish to exfoliate more than once a week.

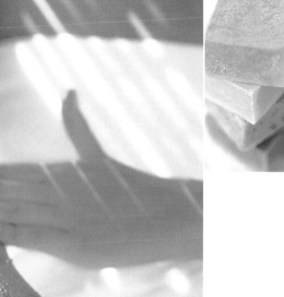
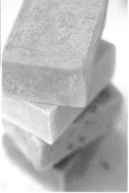

2 tbsp cornmeal

2 tbsp oatmeal

2 tbsp wheatgerm

1 tbsp water

Mix all dry ingredients together and store in an airtight jar. When you want to use it, remove 1 tbsp from the jar, add water and mix to make a paste. Rub in a gentle circular motion over the body to exfoliate dead skin cells, making the complexion smoother. Rinse off under a warm shower.

FROM LEFT: Exfoliating with the skin-softening sugar scrub; A selection of handmade soaps that are packed with natural goodness.
OPPOSITE: The sensitive skin scrub working its magic.

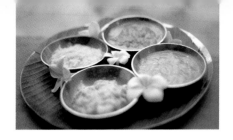

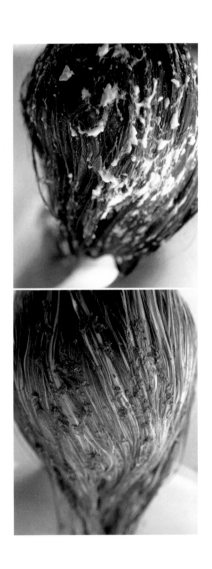

THE HAIR In most cultures, strong, sleek and shiny hair is seen as a sign of beauty. Traditionally, in Asia especially, coconut oil is the shampoo of choice and was used long before modern products became available. Head massage used to be an essential part of hair care, especially among Indian women, who believe that regular head massage with natural vegetable oils keeps their hair healthy, vibrant and really strong.

While hair type and volume are genetic, overall hair condition is personal. Crash diets and high-fat, processed foods are detrimental to hair health, and medication such as the contraceptive pill and diet pills, sleeping tablets and even some cold remedies can make hair dull, brittle and lifeless.

Natural hair colour is determined by melanin, the same pigment that colours the skin. Melanin also helps hair retain its moisture and protect it from sun damage. Grey hair is really a combination of white hair with normal colour, resulting from a reduction in melanin production at the root of the hair follicle. Reduced melanin supply may be genetic but lifestyle factors such as inadequate diet, cigarette smoke and stress also contribute.

While the *Balancing Senses* 10-Day Detox (see page 38–41) cleans the hair from within, the following foods will also help keep hair healthy, shiny and really strong.

- Fruit and vegetables such as blackberries, strawberries, raspberries, grapes, papayas, plums, tangerines, soya beans, carrots, celery, chives, fennel, leafy vegetables like spinach, cabbage and bok choi, onions, parsnips, pumpkins, sweet potatoes and squash.
- Grains, nuts and seeds such as black sesame seeds, oats, brown rice, whole wheat, wheatgerm, pumpkin and flaxseeds, walnuts, almonds and cashew nuts.
- Proteins that are found in lean meat, fish, chicken, eggs and kidneys.
- Herbs including coriander, cinnamon, cloves, ginger and Chinese schizandra or wolfberry, which offers excellent protection against premature greying and hair loss.
- Water—at least 1 L / 1¾ pints per day.

BE SHOPPING SAVVY: HAIR
Although specific hair products and treatments can improve overall texture and condition, some contain harsh stripping agents that can do more harm than good. As with skincare, scan labels before buying products and avoid the ingredients listed on page 91. The key to maintaining a healthy head of hair is ensuring the roots and follicles are well nourished from within. Choose according to your hair type.
OILY HAIR OR SCALP Lime and lemon essential oils can help to reduce oil production. If prone to acne, keep styling products, such as gels, mousse or hair sprays, away from the forehead to avoid clogging of the pores.
DRY HAIR OR SCALP Lavender and geranium essential oils help moisturize, while jojoba, avocado, olive and coconut oils are classic dry hair treatments. Keep your hairdryer on the cool setting to avoid over-drying the hair.

HAIR AND THE SUN Although the sun's rays lighten hair, giving it a healthy sun-kissed glow, they also burn and weaken the hair's protein structure, thereby reducing its elasticity and causing it to break more easily. Chlorine and salt water weaken hair even more. Just as skin is protected from sun damage, so too should hair. Sun protection sprays and leave-in

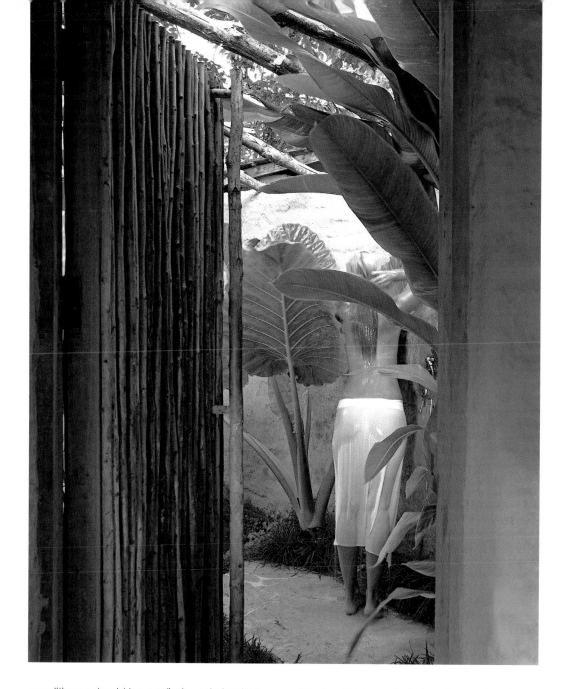

NOURISH YOUR HAIR

- Daily shampooing and conditioning add moisture and shine while also exercising the scalp muscles and encouraging faster and healthier growth.
- Wear a hat or scarf to protect the hair in extreme weather conditions.
- If living in a warm climate or swimming regularly, use a weekly pre-shampoo deep conditioner to protect your hair—see Summer Conditioning Treatment below.
- Guard against split ends by avoiding overbrushing. Brush hair gently and slowly with a blunt comb or a brush with long, widely spaced, plastic bristles.
- Wash your hairbrush and comb weekly by soaking in water with a few drops of tea tree essential oil.
- Caffeine in coffee, tea and soft drinks dehydrates the hair, so consumption is best reduced or avoided altogether.

conditioners should be applied regularly when exposed to the sun. When swimming, mix some waterproof suntan oil with a thick leave-in conditioner and apply in sections along the length of the hair. Comb through for even distribution. Together, the oil and conditioner protect hair from chlorine and sea salt while also conditioning and maintaining moisture. For best results, reapply after swimming.

SUMMER CONDITIONING TREATMENT

This is a weekly pre-shampoo conditioning treatment that nourishes and moisturizes hair from the roots, keeping it healthy and shiny.

2 eggs
2 tbsp olive oil
½ ripe avocado
50 ml / 2 fl oz water

Simply whisk ingredients together and work mixture into the hair with your fingertips. Leave for 10 minutes before shampooing as normal.

BANANA HAIR MASK

1 ripe banana, to revitalize
1 tbsp olive oil, to add shine

Mash the banana in a small bowl and add the olive oil. Using your hands, and with gentle circular massage movements, apply the mixture to the scalp working towards the roots. Cover with a shower cap and hot towel that's been heated when slightly damp in the microwave. Relax for 30 minutes then rinse with warm water. Shampoo and condition as normal. If only the scalp is dry and not the hair, concentrate on applying the mixture to the scalp only, and vice versa.

THICKENING MASK

3–5 celery sticks
2 eggs, free range if available

Juice celery sticks and put aside. Whisk eggs in a bowl. Massage the eggs into your hair and leave in place for 10 minutes. Rinse. Massage the celery juice into your scalp. Leave for 10 minutes and rinse thoroughly. Shampoo and condition as normal.

DANDRUFF DEFYING MASK

For this treatment just mix a large handful of crushed mint leaves into your daily conditioner. Massage into the scalp and leave on your hair for 15–20 minutes. Once the goodness has soaked in, rinse with warm water and shampoo and condition as normal. The ingredients soothe the scalp and prevent flaky skin.

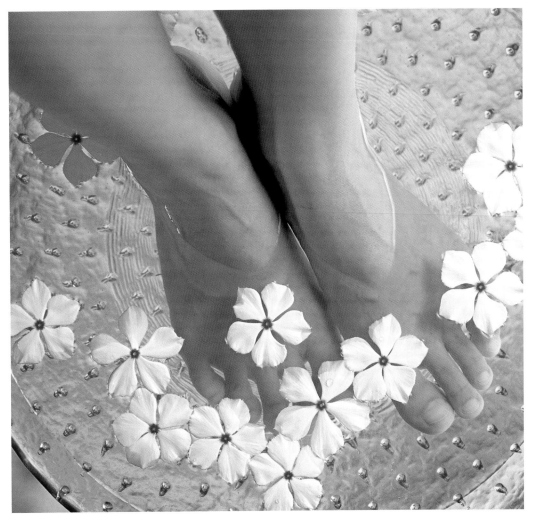

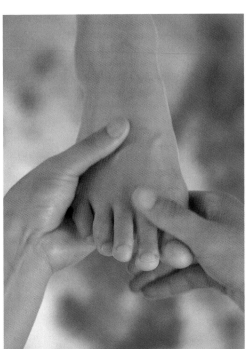

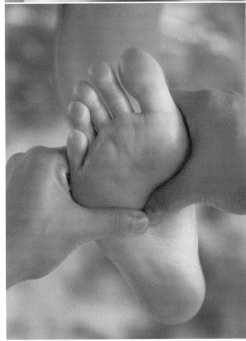

HANDS AND FEET Manicures and pedicures help nails look better, but they need nurturing from within. This is possible with an emphasis on lean meats, eggs, oily fish—like sardines and herrings—dairy products and green leafy vegetables. The nail is about 16 per cent water, so fluid intake is essential for sturdy, strong nails. Also, nails are less porous and absorbent than skin, and they lose moisture a lot faster so a daily moisturizing massage helps stimulate circulation and strengthens the nail bed.

FEED YOUR HANDS, FEET AND NAILS The following foods are ideal for healthy looking hands, feet and nails. FRUIT, NUTS AND SEEDS Blackberries, chestnuts, papaya, peaches, pears, pumpkin, red grapes, strawberries, tangerines, walnuts, sesame and flaxseeds.

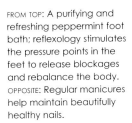

FROM TOP: A purifying and refreshing peppermint foot bath; reflexology stimulates the pressure points in the feet to release blockages and rebalance the body.
OPPOSITE: Regular manicures help maintain beautifully healthy nails.

VEGETABLES Asparagus, soya beans, green leafy vegetables such as spinach, cabbage and bok choi, broccoli, carrots, celery, chives, fennel, green and red beans, kale, mushrooms, onions, parsnips, red capsicums, snow peas, tomatoes, watercress, squash and shallots.

HERBS AND SPICES Coriander, chives, cinnamon, cloves, garlic, ginger, ginseng, wheatgrass and ginkgo biloba.

OTHER FOODS Eggs, chicken, lamb, pork, oysters, oily fish and lean meat.

WATER Drink at least 1 litre / 1¾ pints per day to keep hands, feet and nails healthy.

TO MAINTAIN BEAUTIFUL HANDS AND NAILS

- Always wear gloves when doing your daily housework or DIY projects to protect the skin from harsh cleaning products or abrasive materials that can damage the skin.
- Rub white iodine on the nails with cotton wool to make them stronger; be careful not to use regular iodine as it will stain.
- Gently erase calluses and rough edges on heels and soles of the feet with a damp pumice stone after a bath or shower.
- Allow the feet to breathe naturally by going barefoot as often as possible.
- Indulge in a manicure and pedicure whenever you can.
- Avoid nail polishes that contain formaldehyde and toluene as they can be toxic to the skin that surrounds the nails.
- The skin around the cuticles needs daily nourishment; use a rich cream or lotion and look for one that contains essential oils of lavender and geranium.
- When applying lip balm, rub a little into the cuticles, too, to keep them soft and pliable.

PEPPERMINT FOOT BATH

Water to fill a large bowl, in which to soak feet

1 tsp almond oil

2 drops of peppermint essential oil

Fill the bowl with warm water and add the almond and peppermint oils. Mix the ingredients to disperse, place feet in the bowl and soak for up to 10 minutes. This is ideally done in conjunction with a face and hair mask for some real home therapy. When your feet feel cool, remove them from the bowl. Rinse and dry with a soft towel. This footbath is also a great natural remedy for reducing headaches.

PEPPERMINT FOOT SCRUB

This recipe works to exfoliate the feet and remove hard and dry skin, leaving them feeling fresher and smoother.

2 tbsp almond oil

3 drops rosemary essential oil

3 drops peppermint essential oil

3 tbsp oatmeal, sea salt or shredded natural coconut flesh

Combine almond oil, rosemary and peppermint essential oils in a bowl. Slowly stir in the oatmeal, sea salt or shredded coconut flesh. Apply the mixture in slow, gentle circular movements to the soles of the feet. Leave on the skin for a few minutes then rinse and dry feet with a soft towel.

CITRUS HAND SOAK

450 ml / 16 fl oz warm water

1 tbsp milk

1 tsp baking soda

Fill a bowl with enough water to soak your hands in. Add milk and baking soda and soak hands for 5 minutes. Remove from the bowl, rinse and dry.

AVOCADO HAND REJUVENATOR Use recipe for Avocado Face Mask (see page 94).

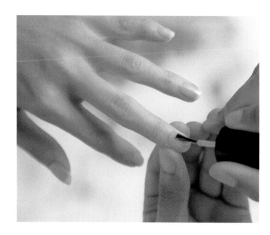

TRADITIONAL CHINESE PALMISTRY

Traditional Chinese palmistry, or the study of the surface of the hands and wrists, is a deeply rooted diagnostic tool in Chinese medicine. Just as reflexology maps the body through the feet, palmistry does the same, but through the hands. Combining age-old wisdom with modern scientific interpretation has led to a deeper understanding of the relationship between the appearance and lines on the hand and disease prevention.

In traditional palmistry the appearance of the hands is said to reveal a person's past, present and future. Through this, practitioners can gain insight into a person's mind, their physical disposition, their emotions and thoughts. Each of the five fingers reflects a person's health at different stages in their life. The thumb reflects childhood; the index finger, youth; middle finger, adulthood; ring finger, later adult life and the little finger, health in old age. When all five fingers are strong with good development and the fingertips are red or ruddy this is a sure sign of healthy blood and energy circulation.

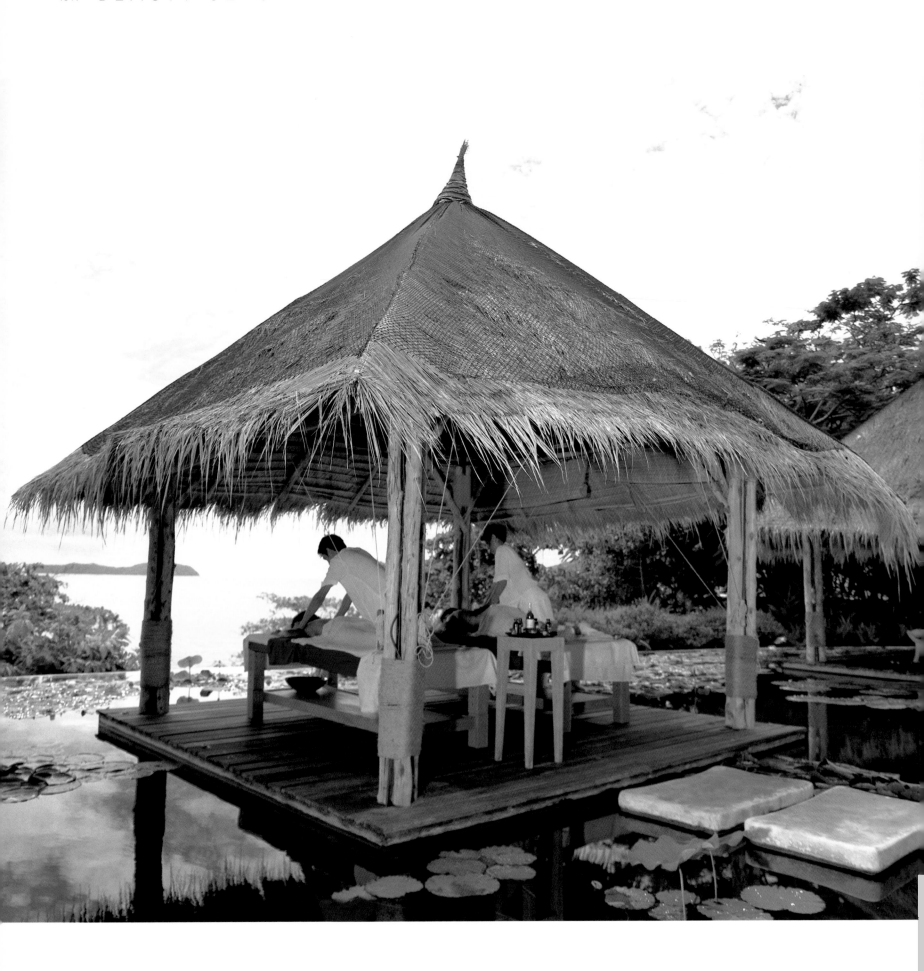

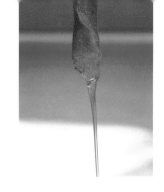

BODY THERAPIES

Around the world, massage is a part of our everyday life since the day we are born. The sense of touch heals the emotions as well as the body. Believed to have originated in Asia as a method of unlocking stagnant *qi*, massage has become the backbone of health and well-being in countries far beyond its roots. And the real beauty of massage as we know it today is that the recipient can benefit from a number of healing traditions within a single treatment. So wherever in the world we may be, from Bombay to Bali, New York to London, we benefit from ancient time-honoured traditions that have been combined with modern scientific techniques to de-stress, heal and truly calm the body, mind and spirit.

Around the globe, therapists guide their hands, and often feet, over client's bodies to ease knots and tension, massaging to calm mind and body. It's no mystery—just the simple power of touch through kneading, stroking, pressing, rubbing and gliding hands, or sometimes arms or other parts of the body, that has proven to unleash countless benefits. These include easing stress, lowering blood pressure, helping stimulate small children, and pure unadulterated pleasure. The following is a taste of these therapies.

INDIAN STYLE MASSAGE

AYURVEDIC MASSAGE Traditional ayurvedic massage combines medicated herbal oils with manual techniques that are aimed at loosening and eliminating the excess *doshas*. It is also administered to enhance circulation, increase flexibility and relieve pain and stiffness. For enhanced healing and pleasure, two therapists can work together in perfect synchrony in a style called *abhyanga*. For the relief of very stubborn aches, the therapist might perform *chavutti pizhichil*, a procedure where he suspends himself by a rope from the ceiling to apply the extra pressure with his feet to undo extreme tension. Ayurvedic massage can also be combined with *shirodhara*.

SHIRODHARA Uniquely ayurvedic, *shirodhara* (massage of the third eye) involves the pouring of a slow, steady stream of warmed medicated oil directly over the third eye, which is located on the brow chakra area. It is a powerful therapy designed to completely relieve mental tension, thereby inducing a calmer and more centred mind.

CHINESE STYLE MASSAGE

ACUPRESSURE Acupressure is a term encompassing a wide range of techniques all of which are based on applying manual pressure to stimulate acupoints in the face and body. This results in regulating and balancing the flow of energy around the body and restoring internal harmony.

REFLEXOLOGY In Chinese thinking, reflex points on the feet correspond to every organ and gland in the body. A skilled reflexologist uses thumb pressure to press and deeply massage each of the tiny reflex zones in the feet to activate the body's natural healing mechanisms. For example, the big toe is connected to the head and simply manually stimulating it eases headaches and tension. The technique has been shown to help relax the body and treat a wide range of acute and chronic conditions from post-natal depression to constipation, diarrhoea, insomnia, back and muscle pain and skin problems.

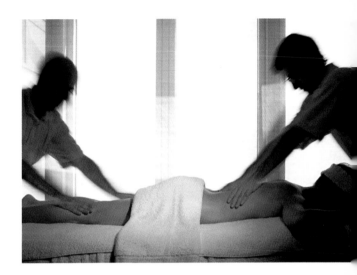

FROM TOP: A constant stream of warm oil is the basis of the unique *shirodhara* treatment; Traditional ayurvedic body massage with two therapists using medicated herbal oils. OPPOSITE: A couple's massage treatment in the sala, close to nature.

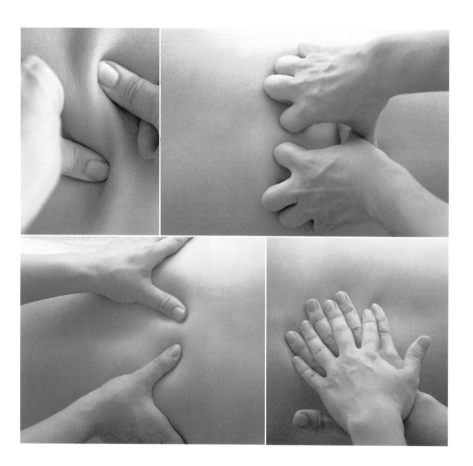

between the thumb and forefinger to spark the nerve endings and stimulate the flow of blood and energy. Other Indonesian massages include *urut*, an intense oil massage based on the meridians and acupoints, and *pijat*, a gentler massage. All are used to re-awaken the body and induce complete relaxation.

SHIATSU Although originally developed in Japan, shiatsu as we know it is a marriage between Chinese acupressure and Western massage techniques that uses a variety of hands-on movements such as holding, pressing and, when appropriate, more dynamic rotations and stretches. All work to improve the flow of vital energy through the body. A distinguishing feature of shiatsu—unlike other physical therapies—is that, by manipulating the body's acupoints, it works on the body's energy system as a whole while being tailored to individual concerns, whether it be back pain, migraine, neck or sports injuries, asthmatic, hormonal or arthritic issues.

SWEDISH MASSAGE Swedish massage is the most popular of all the traditional European massage styles. Developed in the 1700s by Per Henrik Ling—a medical-gymnastic practitioner, who merged Western and Eastern healing techniques—it was the first organized and systematic method of modern therapeutic massage in the Western world. With oil as lubricant, original Swedish massage uses a combination of touching, kneading, rubbing, tapping, and shaking techniques—always made in the direction of the heart—to break down adhesions, relieve pain, clear toxins and relax aching muscles, stimulate the circulation and eliminate toxins.

Shiatsu uses a range of hands-on movements to improve the flow of energy through the body.
OPPOSITE: Massage with Turkey's turquoise coast as a spectacular backdrop at the Six Senses Spa, Bodrum.

TUI NA Literally translated as press and rub, *tui na* involves deep digital stimulation of vital points along the meridians and is the oldest and most common form of Chinese acupressure massage. Using more than 20 different techniques, *tui na* is best used for relieving colds and headaches, insomnia, intestinal upsets, menstrual irregularities, low back pain and stiff neck.

INDONESIAN MASSAGE Traditional Balinese massage is a seamless blend of long sensual strokes combined with acupressure and skin rolling, where the skin is rolled

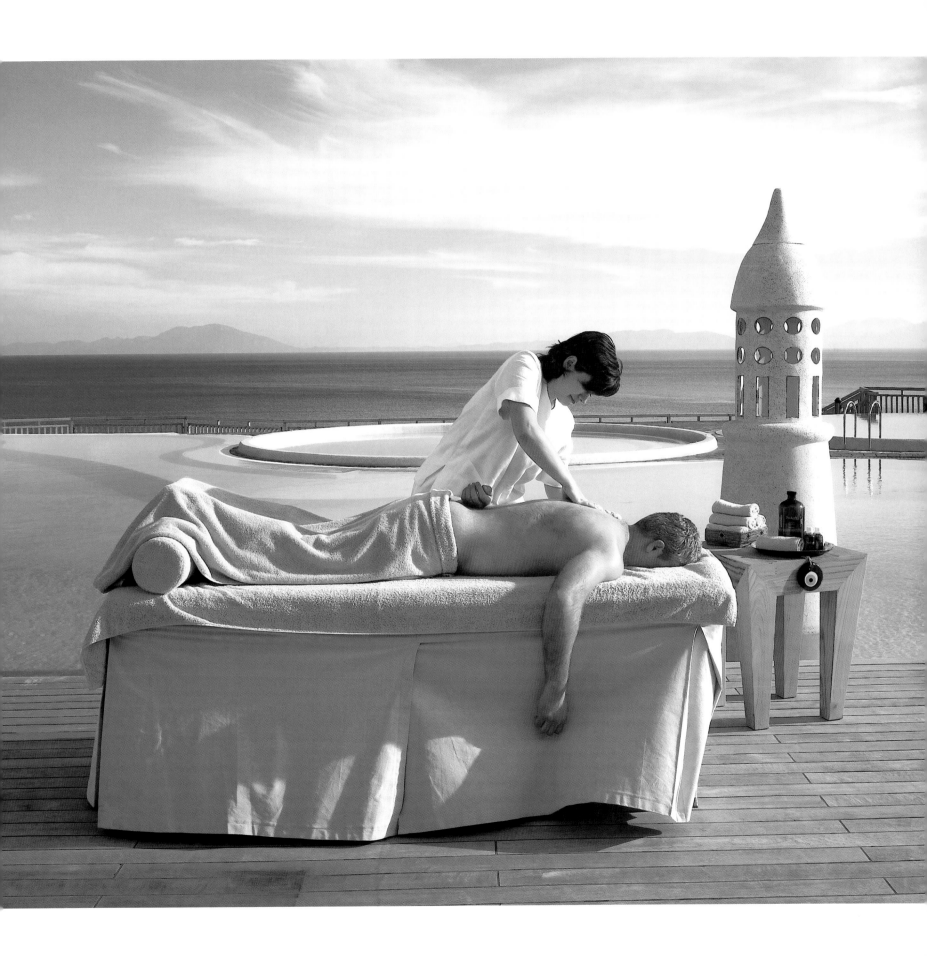

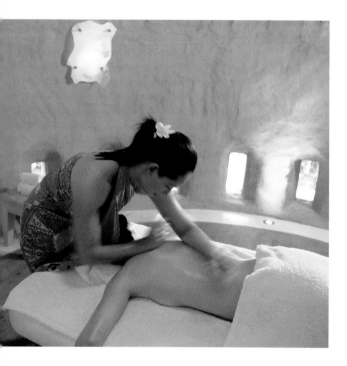

SPORTS MASSAGE
Essentially a form of Swedish massage catering specifically to athletes, sports massage is a central component of a competitive athlete's training regime. It can also help speed up recovery from injury. Sports massage is deliberate and thorough as the therapist must first identify the overused muscles, which are normally hard and tense compared to the surrounding tissues. Then, using specific techniques, knots are loosened and tension is eased completely.

LYMPHATIC DRAINAGE MASSAGE
This gentle technique uses subtle manual manoeuvres to stimulate calm wave-like movements through the lymphatic system to remove toxic build-up and enhance the flow of lymph, the milky fluid in which the organs and muscles are bathed. Working in tandem with the immune system, lymphatic drainage massage helps reduce water retention and clear toxins, making it a perfect prescription for slimming, while also helping relieve sports injuries and body strains.

LOMI LOMI
An utterly uplifting experience, the ancient Hawaiian tradition of Lomi Lomi comes alive with essential oils and rhythmic dance-like massage movements of the palms, knuckles and forearms of one or two therapists in perfect synchrony to disperse stagnant energy, improve circulation and totally revive both body and mind.

STONE THERAPY
Better at retaining hot and cold temperatures than the hands, ultra-smooth stones are increasingly being used in massage. In conjunction with Swedish, Lomi Lomi or other massage styles, the stones give a deeper, more powerful massage workout. It was American therapist Mary Nelson who first used stones in massage. They were heated and anointed with sensual aromas and placed at key chakra points along the body while a soothing massage was administered to relieve pain and restore vitality. As the therapy grew in popularity it developed variations and today heated and chilled stones are commonly used simultaneously with Swedish massage techniques. It's believed the combination gives an added boost to circulation and enhances the body's self-healing. Basalt is most commonly used for the stones, which derive from lava and are shaped and smoothened by nature. Smaller stones are used in facial treatments, reflexology, manicures and pedicures.

AROMATHERAPY MASSAGE AND ESSENTIAL OILS
Essential oils are the aromatic essences extracted from plants, flowers, trees, fruit, bark, grasses and seeds. Each essential oil may contain over 100 components, which, when combined together, exert powerful effects on the body, mind and emotions as they penetrate the bloodstream and infuse their target organs.

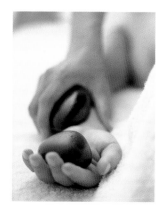

FROM LEFT: Traditional Lomi Lomi massage; Hot stones resting on the palms during a stone therapy massage. OPPOSITE: An uplifting back massage to soothe away aches and pains.

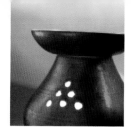

When used in massage, essential oils are carried to the muscle tissue, joints and organs. That's why they complement one another so beautifully, each helping the other, with the ultimate benefit being physical and emotional well-being. While more concentrated oils can be used for the relief of physical complaints like muscle aches and skin lesions—lavender, for instance, helps relieve burns and scarring— essential oils are best diluted with a base oil, such as almond, walnut or evening primrose, before use. This dilution is important especially for sensitive skin or during pregnancy.

Although the Egyptians have a rich history of using aromatic plants as perfumes, credit for aromatherapy as we know it belongs to the French chemist Rene-Maurice Gattefosse. After a lab explosion in his family's perfumery, he plunged his severely burned hand into a container of lavender oil and was amazed at how quickly it healed. From that point his life was devoted to the study of essential oils and their medicinal qualities. Building upon Gattefosse's aromatherapy principles, Madame Marguerite Maury introduced the therapeutic and cosmetic benefits of aromatics in massage during the 1950s.

Over 150 essential oils have been identified to date which can be used alone—for example, a few drops of lavender on the pillow before going to bed to encourage sounder sleep—or in a blend of up to three oils. No more than three should be used, or the individual qualities of the oils will be lost. While a skilled aromatherapist will truly understand their properties, it is generally possible to treat common ailments in the home with some of the more commonly used essential oils. Refer to the chart on the following page.

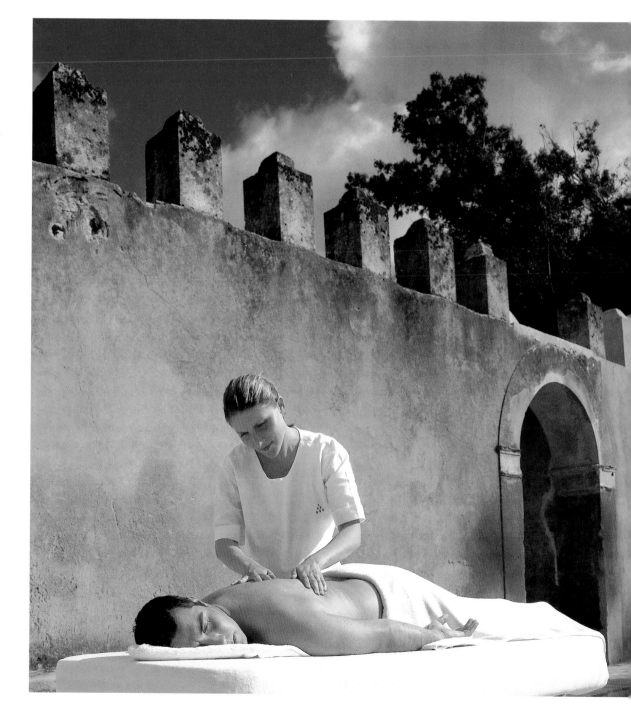

WHEN USING ESSENTIAL OILS BE AWARE OF THE FOLLOWING

- Never take internally.
- Keep essential oils away from the eyes.
- Read about the oil before applying it.
- Essential oils are very concentrated substances and must be diluted before applying directly to the skin. Use a 3 per cent dilution; 3 drops of essential oil for every 100 drops / 1 tsp carrier oil.
- Do not use essential oils with infants. When using with children always use 1 per cent dilution; 1 drop of essential oil for every 100 drops / 1 tsp of carrier oil or water.
- Good carrier oils are sweet almond, grapeseed or sesame seed oils. Unperfumed vegetable oils such as soya or sunflower oil are also appropriate.
- Essential oils are not soluble in water. Make sure you dilute or fully disperse them when using water as a base.
- Essential oils can cause a prickly, irritating sensation on the skin. If this happens, apply vegetable or carrier oil to the irritated area; this will cause the essential oil to be absorbed and will ease the irritation in minutes.
- If skin irritation or an allergic reaction occurs, discontinue use immediately.
- Essential oils should not replace proper healthcare. If you are under medical supervision, consult your healthcare provider before using essential oils.

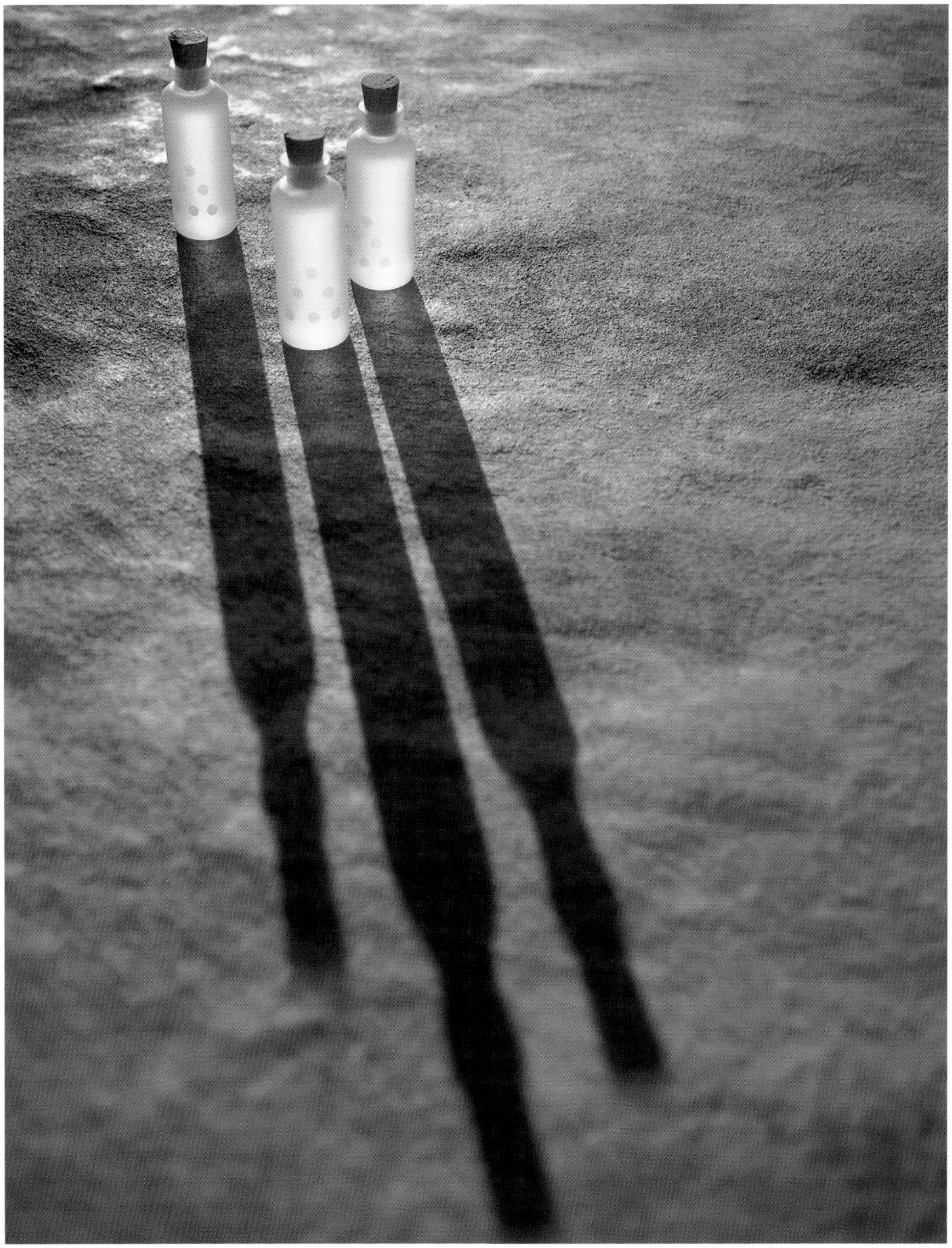

Essential oils can be used in your everyday skincare products—simply add to fragrance-free creams and lotions. Choose according to need and skin type by using the chart opposite.

ESSENTIAL OIL	BENEFITS	TREATS	BLEND WITH
Clary Sage	Awareness: Opens the mind	Reduces sebum production and dandruff. Muscle relaxant, eases stress and tension.	geranium, lavender, marjoram
Geranium	Awareness: Calms the psyche Empowerment: Balances the mind Vitality: Refreshes the mind	Treats inflamed or irritated skin such as acne, eczema and shingles. An antiseptic and astringent, it balances sebum production. A diuretic, it relieves fluid retention and swollen ankles and it is widely known as an antidepressant.	clary sage, lavender, marjoram, cedarwood bergamot, cypress, frankincense
Lavender	Awareness: Brings feelings under control Empowerment: Strengthens the mind	Stimulates and detoxifies skin, helps acne and fluid retention. Offers pain relief, relieves yeast infections, colds and flu. An antiseptic.	clary sage, marjoram, geranium, cedarwood
Marjoram	Awareness: Dispels agitation, warms emotions	Relaxes the muscles. Treats sinus congestion. Prevents intestinal cramps, and lowers blood pressure. Stimulates menstruation, so pregnant women should avoid it.	clary sage, geranium, lavender
Cedarwood	Empowerment: Clears mind, gives strength and harmony	Strengthens hair, detoxifies scalp and hair roots. Its diuretic properties help urinary infections. An antiseptic and expectorant.	geranium, lavender
Juniper	Purpose: Cleanses the mind	Astringent and antiseptic properties make it an excellent tonic for acne. Treats dermatitis, eczema and problems with urino-genital tract.	pine, tea tree
Pine	Purpose: Reactivates energy	Inhaled, it treats respiratory infections such as bronchitis, coughs, colds and sore throats. Helps relieve muscular pain.	juniper, tea tree
Tea Tree	Purpose: Clarifies the mind	Treats respiratory disorders like asthma and bronchitis. Cleanses deeply, helps skin complaints such as acne and rashes. An antiseptic with antiviral, fungicidal properties and helps fight dandruff.	juniper, pine
Myrrh	Self: Amplifies strength and awakens an awareness of spirituality	Helps heal cracked and chapped skin. A soothing antiseptic, it helps relieve sore gums and mouth ulcers. Helps regulate menstrual cycle and ease menstrual pain. Used to ease anxiety and balance emotions.	neroli, vetiver, ylang ylang
Neroli	Self: Assists with confidence	A regenerative oil that treats ageing skin of all skin types. Helps broken veins, and sensitive and inflamed skin. Also a carminative.	myrrh, vetiver, ylang ylang
Vetiver	Self: Protects against oversensitivity	Ideal for ageing or tired skin. A grounding and strengthening essential oil, it can ease extreme nervousness and stress.	myrrh, neroli, ylang ylang
Ylang Ylang	Self: Soothes frustrations, reduces introversion, promotes confidence	Nourishing and moisturizing, for oily, ageing or stressed skin. An antiseptic. Helps lower high blood pressure and slow rapid heartbeat.	myrrh, neroli, vetiver
Basil	Serenity: Relieves mental fatigue	A remedy for liver problems such as headaches and migraines. Inhaled, it eases sinus congestion. Reduces cramps and flatulence. Basil stimulates menstruation, so pregnant women should avoid it.	lemongrass, patchouli, sandalwood
Lemongrass	Serenity: Refreshes the mind	A powerful antiseptic. Relieves headaches when diluted in carrier oil and massaged into the temples. In a footbath, refreshes aching feet. Can irritate the skin; always dilute in carrier oil before use.	basil, patchouli, sandalwood
Patchouli	Serenity: Has sedative effects	An anti-inflammatory, fungicide, and antiseptic, it treats acne, cracked skin, fungal infections, eczema and skin allergies. A traditional tonic, insecticide and stimulant as well as a treatment for snake bites.	basil, lemongrass, sandalwood
Sandalwood	Serenity: An aid to meditation	A tonic for itchy and inflamed skin. Eases bronchitis, throat infections, sinusitis and laryngitis and helps cystitis, diarrhoea and gastritis.	basil, lemongrass, patchouli
Bergamot	Vitality: Uplifting and balancing	Increases photosensitivity, don't use in the sun. A digestive and appetite stimulant, it can also relieve fevers and sore throats.	cypress, geranium, frankincense
Cypress	Vitality: Vitalizes the mind	An antiseptic and astringent, it's good for oily skin. A tonic for the circulatory system, it helps treat asthma and coughs. Helps regulate menstrual cycle and treats varicose veins and haemorrhoids.	bergamot, geranium, frankincense
Frankincense	Vitality: Awakens the higher consciousness	An antiseptic and astringent, it helps heal wounds and smoothen stretch marks. It reduces inflammation and eases rheumatism. Also helps to ease stress and anxiety.	bergamot, cypress, geranium

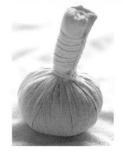

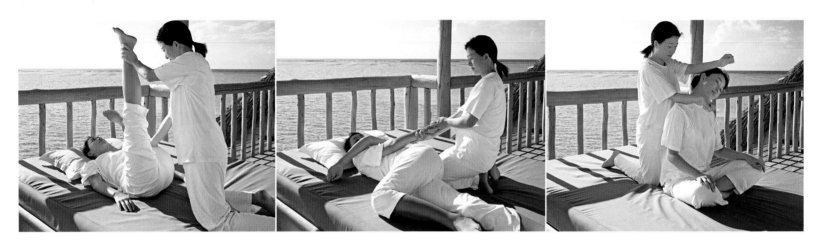

A herbal compress packed with dried herbs; The stretching movements of traditional Thai massage ease tension and promote flexibility through the body. OPPOSITE: No oil is used, rather loose clothing should be worn as the therapist manipulates your body.

THAI MASSAGE Thai massage or *nuat bo'rarn*—meaning ancient massage—is a blend of time-honoured Chinese acupressure techniques with yogic manipulation. This form of massage was originally practised in Buddhist temples exclusively by specialized monks. Today, Thai massage is available around the world, but the monks at Wat Pho in Bangkok still administer massage and pass on their skills.

The authentic Thai experience is performed on a floor mat, both parties wear loose comfortable clothing and it begins with a meditative prayer called a *puja* recited in the original Pali language which reminds the therapist of the *Four Divine States of Mind* according to Buddhist teachings and helps them reach a meditative state. It is said that only when a masseur performs his 'art' in a meditative mood can he be considered a truly good practitioner of Thai massage.

Massage Thai-style combines gentle pressure with the hands and feet using a wide variety of passive stretching movements. The therapist uses his hands, forearms, knees and feet to apply pressure to the *sên* (acupoints), while also pulling, twisting and manipulating

the body to encourage a smoother flow of energy. While it does not necessarily seek to relax the body—unlike most Western massages—to the devoted Thai massage is a dynamic and physical experience that integrates body, mind and spirit and, when performed in a quiet, meditative atmosphere, it loosens the body completely, releasing it of tension and toxic material and thoroughly energizing the system.

THAI HERBAL COMPRESS This authentic style of Thai massage uses local herbs such as turmeric, camphor, lemongrass, kaffir lime and ginger, which are wrapped tightly in muslin cloth. Tied tightly, the compresses are then infused in hot water or steam. The *bolus* (compress) is then used as a massage medium and applied either on specific parts of the body or the whole body. Its warm herbal mixture effectively eases tension, relieves sore muscles and improves the flow of energy. A Thai herbal compress is especially effective for women who have recently given birth as it soothes and calms the muscles and gently eases the mind.

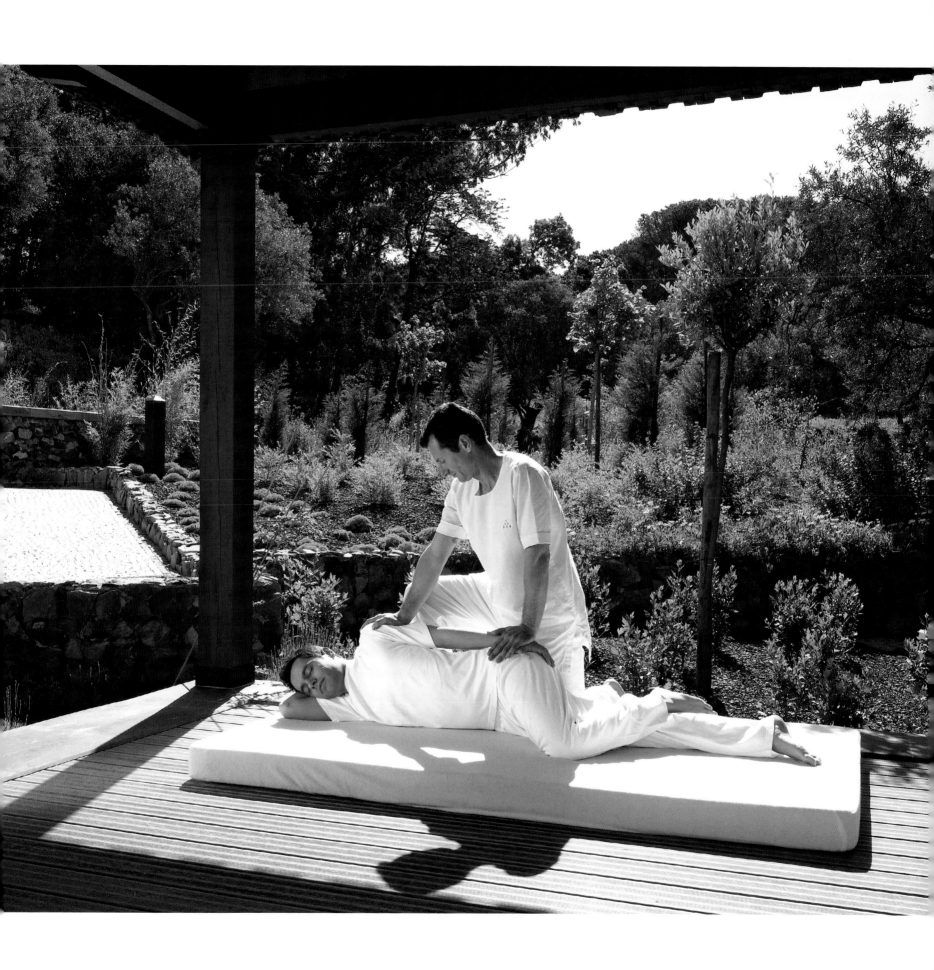

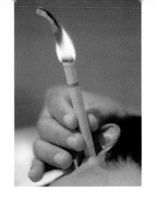

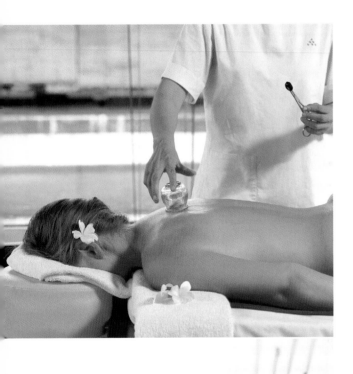

FROM TOP: Ear candling with specific candles that are placed inside the ear to melt wax and cleanse the ear canal; During cupping treatments, suction moves stagnant or blocked energy and rebalances the body; Some acupuncture needles. OPPOSITE: Couples can enjoy their treatments together.

ACUPUNCTURE A popular time-tested and traditionally Chinese method of rebalancing any disrupted energy in the body, acupuncture has recently won many converts in the West. Its one great advantage over Western medicine is that it does absolutely no harm; unlike drugs and surgery it has virtually no side effects.

A skilled acupuncturist inserts needles at specific points along the body's meridians or energy centres, thereby pulsing the body with a low electric current to free blocked energy. Although Western scientists remain sceptical, they know in certain situations it does work because it produces measurable changes in the brain. Normally, most people's response to acupuncture treatment is gradual, with symptoms sometimes worsening before marked improvement is noted.

Acupuncture gained official worldwide recognition in 1979 when the World Health Organization (WHO) issued a list of health conditions deemed appropriate for acupuncture treatment. In this list were stress, headaches and migraines, female fertility problems, pregnancy-induced nausea, menstrual cramps, constipation, ulcers, tennis elbow, insomnia and general muscle pain. Acupuncture can also be used in skincare; it's said to firm and uplift the face and delay the signs of ageing.

MOXABUSTION Moxa is a dried herb more commonly known as mugwort, *Artemisia vulgaris*. The most common form of moxa used today is the moxa stick, a compressed moxa leaf resembling a mini cigar. When lit, the stick is held above the skin to warm the desired acupuncture point and activate the energy

channels. Moxabustion can be used alone, as part of an acupressure massage, or it can be combined with acupuncture where the herbs are burnt on the end of inserted needles. However it is administered, moxa relieves muscular problems, sports injuries and some stress-related complaints.

CUPPING An ancient form of Chinese therapeutic massage, cupping now enjoys a cult following with widely photographed tell-tale marks on celebrities' backs. While the ancient Taoists used hollow animal horns or bamboo, experts today use glass bulb-shaped jars which are fixed onto various points on the body. Using a pump to create a vacuum, the suction moves stagnant or blocked *qi* and invigorates the body. Traditionally, a natural vacuum was created by waving a flame beneath the jar immediately before it was placed on the skin. Cupping is successfully used for the relief of arthritic pain and menstrual problems, and is often practised in conjunction with acupuncture and massage.

EAR CANDLING Originally practised by Native American Indians to cleanse and harmonize the aura, ear candling or coning is hugely popular in the West. It's a simple means of cleansing the ear canal and sinus passage and removing blockages. It is also believed to relieve headaches, migraines, ear infections, tinnitus, chronic sinusitis and inner ear pressure.

Specially designed candles, are lit and placed inside the ear to melt earwax and ease pressure. The procedure is utterly painless and completely relaxing, and for most people just 2–3 sessions leaves the ears completely clean and hearing as nature intended.

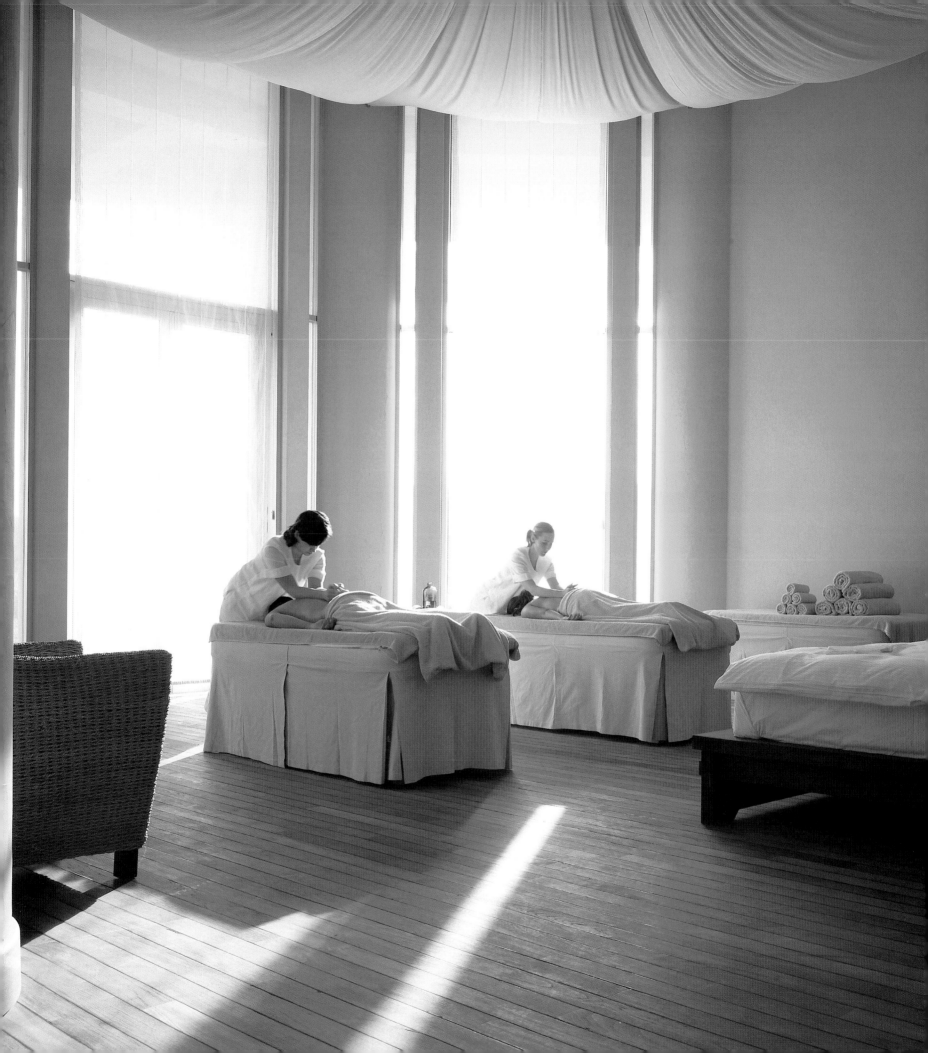

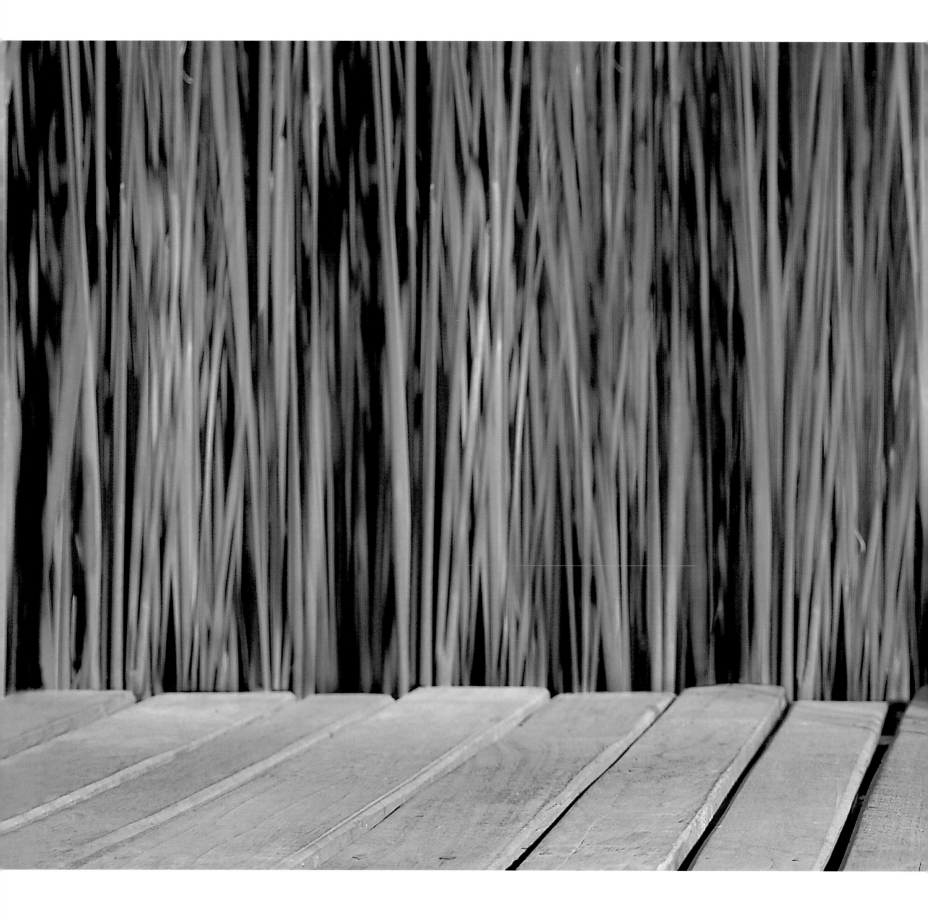

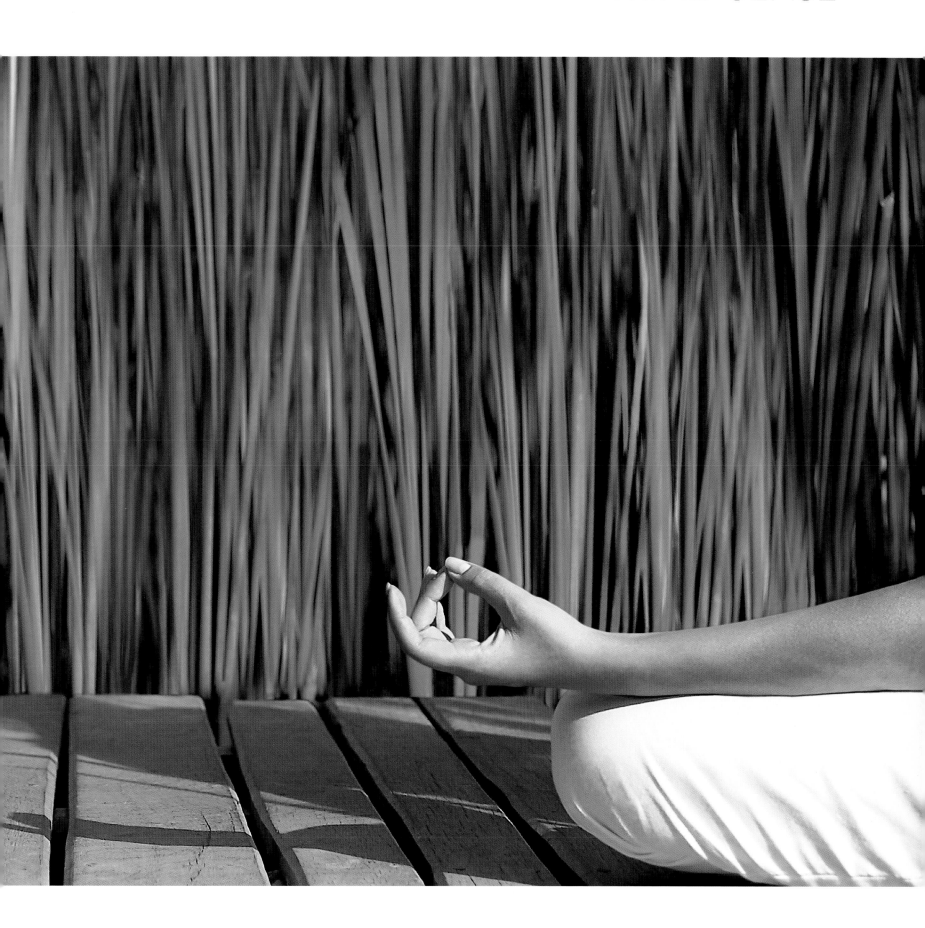

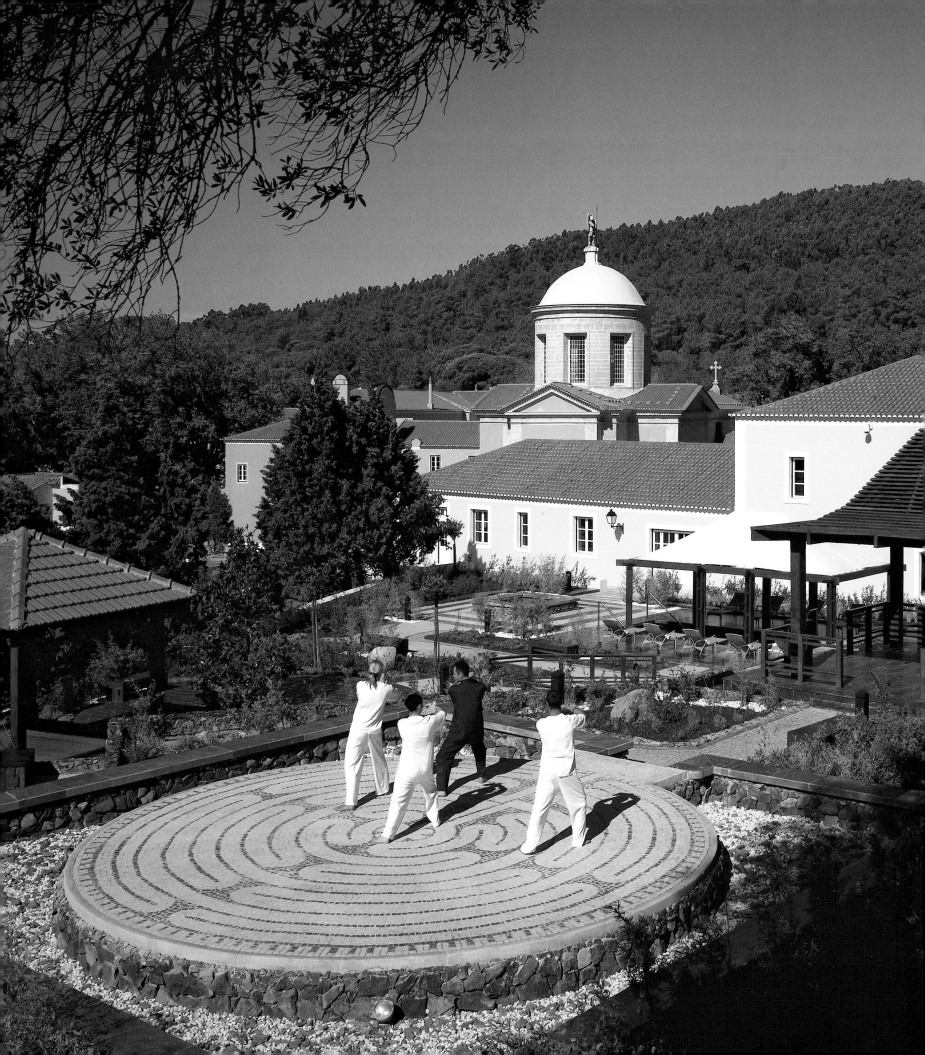

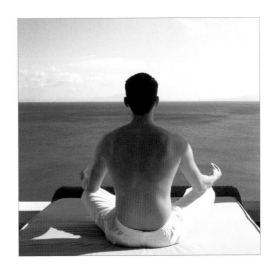

MIND SENSE

When the mind is calm and stable, the vitality of life circulates harmoniously throughout the body. If the body is nourished and protected by this circulation of vitality, how can it possibly become ill?

-Yellow Emperor's *Classic of Internal Medicine* (220BC)

Although time-honoured traditions like traditional Chinese medicine (TCM) and Indian ayurveda offer comprehensive guidelines on achieving mind-body health and well-being, few practices exist that focus exclusively on spiritual health. This may be due to the fact that, unlike body and mind, spirit is not measurable and cannot be studied in isolation. Lives today are so busy, there are more things to do, more goals to achieve, more money to earn and more rewards to reap. However, in spite of this materialistic growth, people are increasingly recognizing the downside and realizing that we are losing sight of who we really are. Each of us has the answers within; it's simply a matter of listening to them and acting on what they tell us. It can be as simple as finding the right key, and spiritually uplifting therapies such as yoga, t'ai chi and meditation help us experience this connection.

Many spas are now reflecting this heightened awareness of spiritual matters by offering an increasing range of programmes based on energy balance and improved self-awareness to help achieve inner calm and a more settled mind. It is the teachings and tenets of Buddhism that form the backbone of many of these programmes. They can be detected by, for example, the mere presence of lotus flowers, of calming rituals such as footbaths, and most notably by the practice of yoga, t'ai chi, *qi gong*, pranayama and meditation, which are fundamental to all mind and spirit wellness philosophies.

As more and more Western medical practitioners embrace the world of wellness, they too appreciate that listening to the voice within may be the answer to many of today's health crises. This is preventive medicine at its best and the heart of TCM and ayurvedic philosophies. Spiritual health means learning to trust our inner voice, recognizing and experiencing our innate potential and enhancing our spiritual potential—all essential components of daily lives that can easily be adopted, adapted and practised. With this self-realization comes a confidence, not easily destroyed.

The perfect spot for some quiet contemplation is a peaceful place where you won't be interrupted. OPPOSITE: The most effective time to practise yoga is as the sun is rising, the body is awakened, ready for the day ahead.

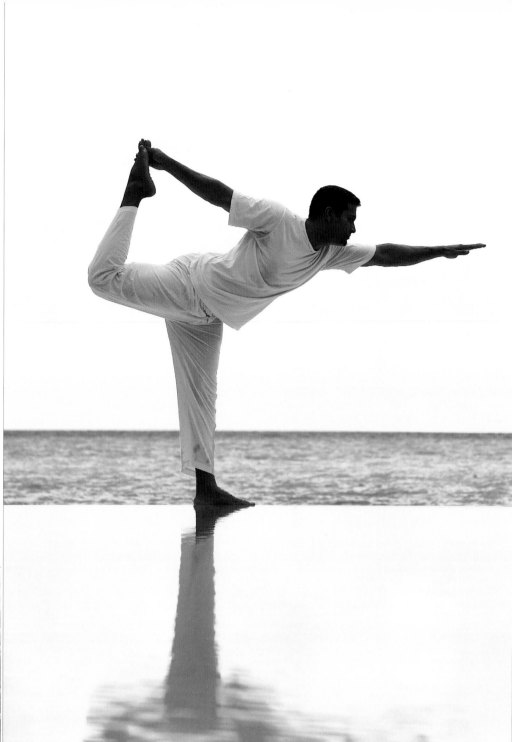

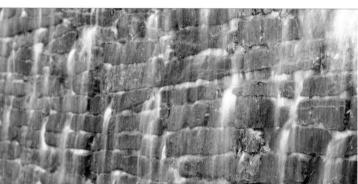

The Lord of the Dance pose that stretches the limbs and builds strength and stability. OPPOSITE: As you lean backwards or clasp your hands together behind your back, the shoulders and chest are opened therefore deepening the breath.

Flowing water never stagnates. The hinges of an active door never rust. This is due to movement. The same principle applies to essence and energy. If the body does not move, *qi* does not flow and energy stagnates.

-*Spring and Autumn Annals* (4BC)

MOVEMENT From the earliest times, ancient scholars recognized the importance of soft, flowing spiritual exercises as essential for cultivating the essence and energy that lie at the root of real health. These are far more subtle forms of exercise than many Western sports, yet they offer a more powerful mind-body workout, leaving you feeling physically and spiritually brighter, stronger and more in tune with your creative and expressive self. They are fast becoming a central part of daily life, helping us live as we were born to.

Regular practice of yoga can help you face the turmoil of life with steadiness and stability.

- BKS Iyengar

YOGA Yoga, the ancient method of body-mind integration originally practised by Hindu sages to help achieve enlightenment, has remained as vibrant and responsive to the changing environment as it was over 5,000 years ago. A Sanskrit word meaning union or joining together, this multi-level discipline ranges from the simple practice of a series of daily exercises called *asanas* to a complete mind, body and spirit philosophy for life incorporating diet, movement and meditation.

Yoga today is no longer guru-oriented or religion-based. It never demands acceptance from any specific belief system. Rather, yoga is a pathway of spiritual enquiry that is open to all, and is awakened by an earnest desire for a deeper understanding of life. Moreover, with the help of its celebrity clientele such as Madonna and Christy Turlington—former runway queen and now one of the most recognized faces of yoga East and West—yoga has become a popular choice for those wanting a strong, supple and healthy body.

Unlike many other forms of exercise, yoga's genius lies in the fact that it is not just a series of physical exercises but it also fulfils a genuine need. That is to find some peace and clarity in an increasingly turbulent and stressful world. Very much like the spa experience today, where people are desperately seeking more than soft skin, the emphasis lies on feeding and nurturing the mind and emotions as well as the body. The purpose is not to escape life but to embrace it more completely and one of its

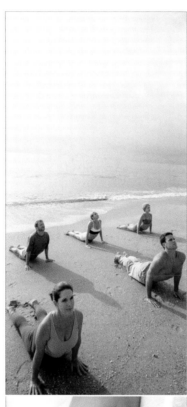

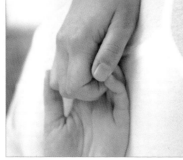

most beautiful facets is its openness and versatility. These important elements allow practitioners to focus on either the physical, psychological or spiritual aspects of yoga—or indeed, a combination of them all.

FOUNDATIONS OF YOGA Although the *Bhagavad Gita* is the earliest complete work on yoga dated around 5BC, much of what is known today is derived from Yoga's classical and seminal text, the *Yoga Sutras* written by an Indian sage, Patanjali, in 3BC. Originally written in Sanskrit, the *Yoga Sutras* discusses many facets of life and offers practical instruction on how to achieve yoga's promises, beginning with a code of conduct for living and ending. This is illustrated by a central character's vision of his true self, which shows the ultimate goal of yoga.

According to the *Yoga Sutras* the science of yoga consists of eight *ashtanga* or limbs—the *yama*, *niyama*, *asana*, pranayama, *pratyahara*, *dharana*, *dhyana* and *samadhi*, see following page. These elements work with the body on both physical and spiritual levels—from *asanas* that relax and tone the muscles and massage the internal organs; to pranayama that controls the breath and regulates the flow of prana; to meditation that ultimately calms and heals the spirit. Each element is beneficial, but when carried out together they comprise the essence of yoga therapy. Some postures are not just physically challenging but mentally demanding as well, as the practice asks you to search for the position through the breath. In doing so, you are brought to the present, time and time again and, as long as you are breathing correctly and working with the breath in each posture, actually awakening the *shakti* or spiritual energy within.

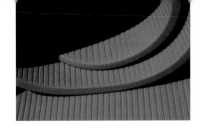

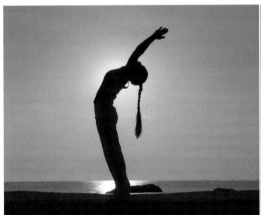 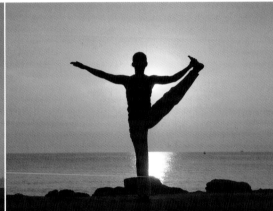 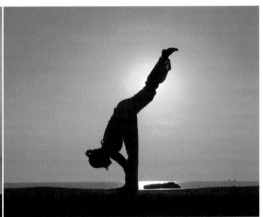

Three poses at different stages of an advanced salute to the sun sequence. OPPOSITE: The warrior pose, also part of a salute to the sun sequence, demands core strength and balance.

Presented in a style known as sutra, with very few words yet universal in context and free from ambiguity, the *Yoga Sutras* links the teacher with the teaching. This fundamental relationship is the essence of yoga practice; in other words, it is the teacher who brings the heart to life. The short but concise words of the original writings have facilitated efficient oral transmission from teacher to student throughout the centuries with many scholars and gurus contributing along the way, making yoga what it is today. Through the help of these teachers, turbulent minds are brought to peace and extraordinary wisdom, and well-being becomes possible.

In our all-consuming world, some argue that the true tradition of yoga is being diluted for commercial benefit and, with the emphasis very much on yoga's physical practice, we are missing out on the most profound benefits that yoga could have on our lives. Perhaps so, but what is important is staying true to the tradition of yoga and through regular practice becoming toned, healthy and more in tune with ourselves in the deep calm that lies beyond the clutter of our clouded minds.

YOGA'S EIGHT LIMBS
- **YAMA**
  The laws of life and attitudes toward the environment, comprising *ahisma*, the Hindu ethic of non-violence, restraint from lying, stealing and greed.
- **NIYAMA**
  Attitudes toward ourselves, comprising cleanliness, serenity, study, devotion and asceticism.
- **ASANA**
  The physical postures.
- **PRANAYAMA**
  Breath control for energizing and balancing the mind-body through the flow of breath and prana.
- **PRATYAHARA**
  Drawing attention to silence and internalization of the senses to activate the mind.
- **DHARANA**
  Concentration and steadiness of mind.
- **DHYANA**
  Meditation and prolonged concentration that fills the consciousness.
- **SAMADHI**
  Ultimate state of self-realization and the settled mind.

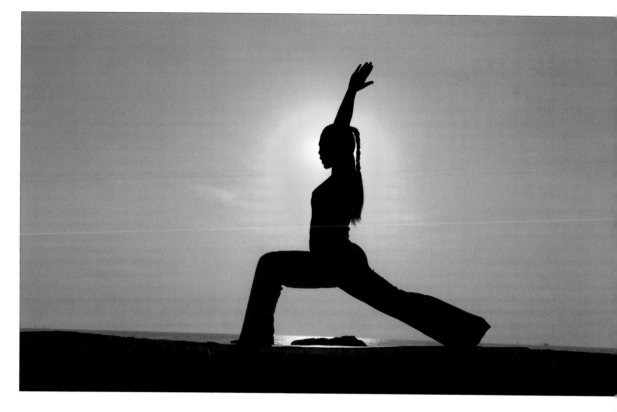

YOGA STYLES While all styles of yoga aim to balance body, mind and spirit, they go about it differently, for example, how the *asanas* are done and where the attention is focused either on mastering the holding of the posture or on breathing or alignment. Some use props, while others crank up the temperature and go for the sweat. No particular style is best. It's down to personal preference and, regardless of the style chosen, yoga is all about you and listening to the voice within. The following is a guide to the more common styles of yoga.

HATHA Many yoga styles are rooted in *hatha*, yoga's physical discipline that focuses on developing control of the body through a series of *asanas* and pranayama or breathing techniques. In Sanskrit, *ha* represents the sun and *tha*, the moon. Much like the yin and yang of TCM, *hatha* represents the duality of life and it leads the way to balancing opposing forces in the body and in life.

ASHTANGA This physically demanding practice was developed by K. Pattabhi Jois to build strength, flexibility, and stamina. Not for the weak-hearted, *ashtanga* yoga offers a fast-paced series of sequential poses beginning with sun salutations. Students move from one posture to another in a continual flow, with movements intimately linked with correct breathing. Power yoga is based on *ashtanga*.

BIKRAM Created by Bikram Choudhury—guru to the stars—this is hot yoga practice with the room temperature of between 29°C–37°C / 85°F–100°F. In this hot and steamy environment, students vigorously perform 26 poses designed to cleanse the body from the inside out.

IYENGAR Developed by B.K.S. Iyengar, this form of yoga stresses a deeper understanding of how the body works. Students focus on symmetry and alignment, using props such as straps, blankets, wooden blocks, and chairs to achieve postures. Each pose is held for a longer time than in most other styles of yoga.

KARMA The *Bhagavad Gita* ascribes a central place to karma yoga, stating that in life we can only act, and we should not be affected by our actions. Emphasizing selfless behaviour, karma states that we must involve ourselves through action, but leave the rest to God and expect nothing. If the fruits of our endeavours do not match our expectations then we should not be disappointed.

KRIPALU The yoga of consciousness or wilful practice was developed by the founder of the Kripalu Centre of Health and Healing, Amrit Desai, in Massachusetts, USA in 1966. Based on the postures of *hatha* yoga, the emphasis in *Kripalu* is on listening to the body for feedback during yoga practice, with the goal being as much psychological as it is physical.

KUNDALINI Once a guarded secret in India, *kundalini* yoga arrived in the West in 1969, when Sikh Yogi Bhajan challenged tradition by teaching it publicly. *Kundalini* mixes chanting and breathing practice with yoga *asanas* that are designed to awaken *kundalini* energy, which is stored at the base of the spine. A Sanskrit word meaning coiled one, *kundalini* is often symbolized by a coiled snake.

RAJA Raja means king, and this yoga path is often called the royal road as it includes all eight limbs of yoga. Raja yoga offers a comprehensive means of controlling the waves of thought by turning the mental and physical energy into spiritual energy with absolute inner control—meditation is a key element.

SIVANANDA Founded by Swami Vishnu-devananda, *sivananda's* gentle approach takes students through the 12 sun salutation postures and incorporates chanting, meditation and deep relaxation. Students are encouraged to embrace a healthy lifestyle and vegetarian diet along with positive thinking and meditation.

TANTRA Routinely misunderstood, tantra is less about sexual indulgence and more about discovering and stimulating sensual spirituality. It works with the *kundalini* energy and teaches practitioners how to use this for sensual pleasure and for bringing joy and wholeness to everyday life. Tantra yoga practice includes visualization, chanting, *asana*, and strong breathing.

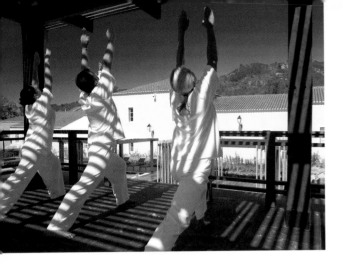

An early morning t'ai chi class to jumpstart the body's flow of energy.
OPPOSITE: T'ai chi movements are intimately linked with animals in nature and help promote inner relaxation and strength.

QI GONG AND T'AI CHI

In Chinese, the word vitality is used to signify a combination of energy, spirit and the vital essence of life that is the basis of health and longevity, and the foundation of immunity and resistance.

Soft flowing exercises such as *qi gong* and t'ai chi that mirror the movement of nature are as much a part of Chinese culture as yin and yang as they circulate *qi* to feed the mind and emotions as well as the body. Originally conceived as a means of fighting disease—in many ancient cultures exercise was an adjunct to medicine—to the Chinese these time-honoured martial arts are a means of focusing the mind and developing inner strength. Central to effective practice is that the movements are soft and smooth and performed in conjunction with deep breathing. This switches the nervous system from a chronically overactive sympathetic mode to a calming, restorative parasympathetic mode in which the body's vital functions and energies are balanced and the secretions of vital essences—such as hormones—are stimulated.

QI GONG Based primarily on movements learned by observing animals in nature, *qi gong* was first mentioned in the earliest written records of Chinese history when it was practised as a therapeutic dance to cure rheumatism. With the current resurgence of Chinese philosophy, this powerful self-healing discipline remains hugely popular and is seen as the most effective guardian and regulator of *qi*.

The literal translation for *qi gong* is energy work, but the actual practice and applications of these flowing movements are far deeper, orchestrating perfect balance and harmony, connecting the body through the breath. There are various forms of *qi gong*, including Buddhist, Taoist, Confucian and martial arts methods, with the main difference being the level of activity involved and where the breath and energy are focused—be it on building inner strength or on cultivating the mind.

While *qi gong* is routinely prescribed across China for the relief of chronic pain, it is also believed to strengthen the body's resistance to disease, reduce blood pressure, harmonize internal body functions, improve posture and muscle tone and, most importantly, bring the body to a state of peace, increasing flexibility, stamina, balance and grace.

T'AI CHI In *T'ai Chi—A Way of Centring and I Ching*, t'ai chi is defined as "*meditation in movement, a philosophical system, a set of principles of self-defence, a prophylaxis against disease, and exquisite dance. It corrects your posture and enhances relaxation. It energizes your body and tranquilizes your spirit. It is a bridge between Eastern meditation and Western psychotherapy, integrating the mind and the senses.*"

Literally translated as supreme ultimate, t'ai chi was originally developed from *qi gong* by blending its internal meditation association with external exercise to further promote inner relaxation and strength. In t'ai chi there are short forms with 64 movements and longer sessions with 108 movements that can be done slowly or quickly. Central to effective practice is developing power and strength, grace and flexibility. All movements share names related to nature such as 'waving hands like clouds' and 'repulsing the monkey', proof that these instinctive movements are linked with the natural world. Indeed, t'ai chi has a rhythm simulating nature, such as a flowing river, and it brings a real sense of peace and serenity.

STANDING POSTURE In ancient times, the standing posture was one of the secrets passed down from the master to a few very select disciples. The original posture has been modified slightly over time, but it is still one of the most efficient methods for mobilizing *qi* in the body. The standing posture is best practised twice a day: first thing in the morning and just before going to bed. While beginners are normally only able to hold the posture for a short time, with time and daily practice you should be able to stand for up to 20 minutes at a stretch.

Stand with the feet parallel and shoulder width apart. Keep the knees loose, not rigid, and hold hands at your side. Slowly bend your knees to squatting. At the same time, raise your hands, palms facing down, to chest height in front of you, until they are parallel to the ground. Look straight ahead with your nose directly in line with your navel. Your neck and shoulders should be relaxed, your arms spread and hands relaxed—but not limp, your back should be erect and legs firmly anchored. When comfortable in this position, close your eyes and focus on your breathing. Breathe in and out slowly, so the abdomen—rather than the chest—expands and contracts with each breath. If you find it hard to focus, then count your breaths up to 10 and repeat. You should soon start to feel the breath flowing through the body and your hands will start to warm. If your hands do not warm, then you are not relaxed enough for the *qi* to flow freely. Keep practising, always ensuring that the shoulders are dropped and relaxed. This sensation of warmth should slowly start to permeate the body until you begin to sweat, which is a sure sign of healthy flowing *qi*.

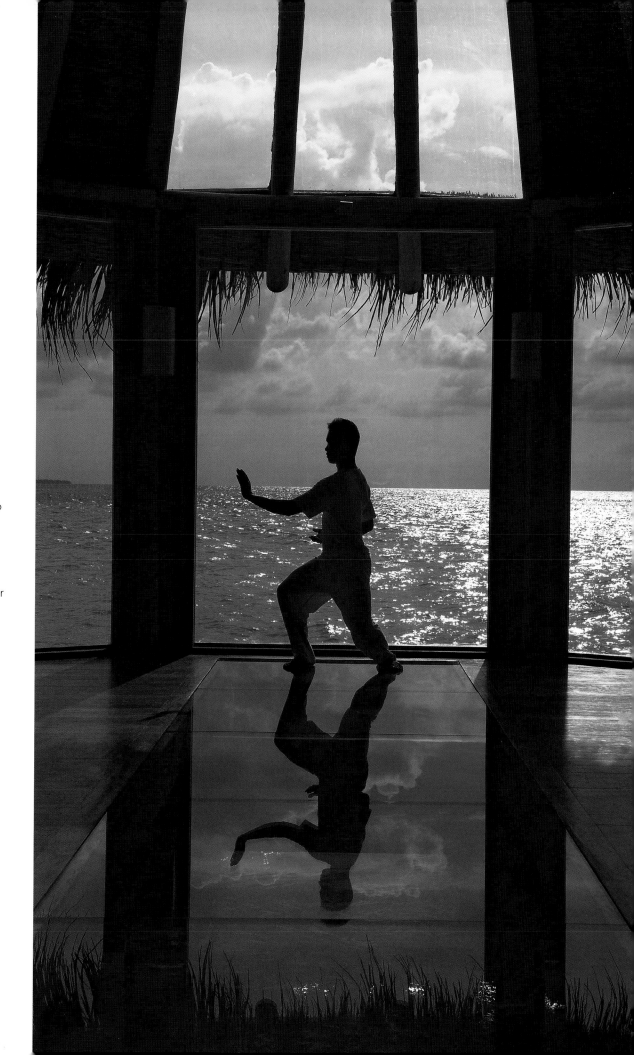

Pranayama is the connecting link between the body and the soul of man, and the hub in the wheel of yoga.

-B.K.S. Iyengar

PRANAYAMA Pranayama, or breath control, is an extensively used technique for harmonizing the flow of prana through the body, and achieving spiritual awareness and well-being. It is as central to yoga as breathing is to living. In Sanskrit, the word prana means both energy and breath, while *yama* means control, discipline or regulation. Together they refer to the prolongation and restraint of the breath. The complex practice of different breathing techniques involves exercises that

have the potential to affect the body both physically and physiologically as well as the body's psychological and cerebral activities such as memory and creativity. Pranayama is credited with conferring on the practitioner a calm, balanced and focused spirit, and increased vitality and longevity.

One of the goals of yoga is to achieve a level of fluidity between the mind, body and spirit. A central tenet to pranayama is that as we can influence the flow of prana through

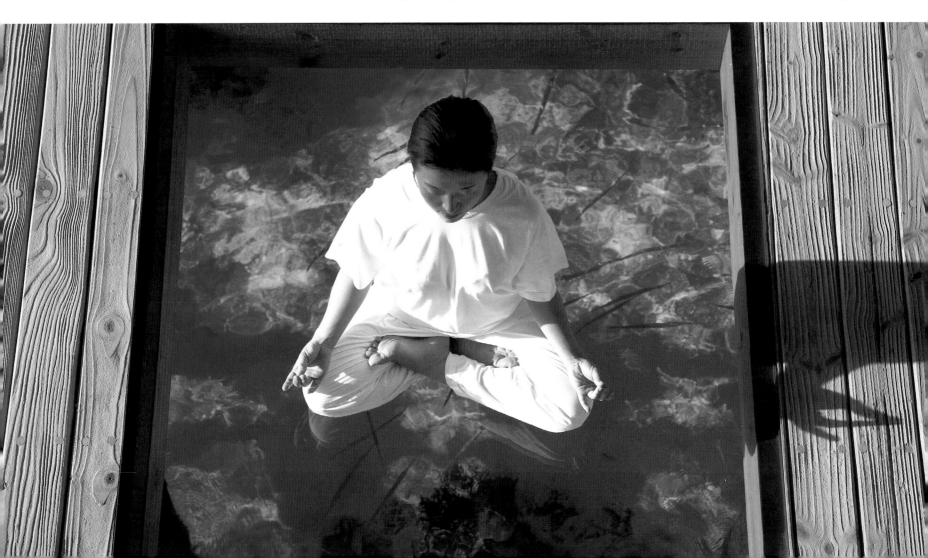

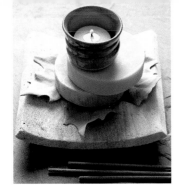

the flow of the breath, therefore the quality of the breath should be carefully considered as it can influence the state of mind. Through yoga and pranayama these connections are maximized and are considered the perfect preparation for the stillness of meditation.

When practising pranayama, it is important to find a sitting position in which you can remain for a lengthy period without feeling sore and stiff. While pranayama techniques are used in certain *asanas* to help the body achieve some of the more demanding positions, in pranayama practice itself, a posture must be adopted that does not disturb the breath and keeps the spine upright at all times. For most people the best positions are lotus or half lotus pose, sitting on a chair with spine erect or even kneeling with the knees tucked underneath or to the sides of the body.

There are various recognized pranayama techniques but one of the most popular is *ujjayi* meaning victorious breath, and known as throat breathing. This is practised during many forms of yoga, especially *ashtanga*. So much so that the sound of deep *ujjayi* breathing during *ashtanga* practice can be quite intimidating, particularly for a beginner. Correct *ujjayi* breathing helps enrich the flow of prana through the body and supports the practitioner during difficult postures while also serving as an internal metronome measuring the duration of postures by the number of breaths held.

Another pranayama technique is *nadi shodhana* or alternate nostril breathing. It cleanses the nasal passages and balances the right and left hemispheres of the brain. Regularly practised at the beginning of an *ashtanga* or meditation class, it clears the mind and awakens the body in preparation for practice.

UJJAYI BREATHING TECHNIQUE

Sit in a comfortable position, like the lotus or half lotus (see page 133), and draw air in slowly but deeply through both nostrils. You should keep the mouth and the back of the throat or glottis partially closed. The larynx is contracted as you breathe, slightly narrowing the air passage, and therefore it produces a soft snoring sound with every breath. This sound should be even and continuous throughout exhalation, with the mouth always closed and with similar volumes of air always being inhaled and exhaled. This breathing technique is commonly used during yoga practice.

NADI SHODHANA BREATHING TECHNIQUE

In this technique both inhalation and exhalation are lengthened. This is achieved by breathing alternately through each nostril while keeping the mouth closed and without using the throat. To begin, sit in a comfortable position, like the lotus or half lotus (see page 133), and hold the right thumb and third finger on the point where the cartilage begins in the nose, which is the narrowest part of the nasal passage. Gently close the right nostril with your thumb and breathe in slowly and smoothly through the left nostril. Hold the breath and close the left nostril with the ring finger. At the same time, lift your thumb opening the right nostril to exhale slowly and evenly. Hold the breath for a few seconds before inhaling again, this time through the right nostril and exhaling through the left. For optimal results repeat this cycle at least five times, slowly building up to 12, with a similar ration of breaths and ensuring breathing between the nostrils is even, smooth and regular. Continuous practice will help balance the left and right hemispheres of the brain. An easy breathing exercise, it can be done anywhere and at anytime.

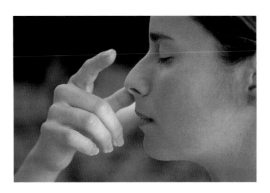

As long as there is breath in the body, there is life. When breath departs, so too does life. So regulate the breath.

- The Hatha Yoga Pradipika

Try meditating while gazing at a lit candle; Alternate nostril breathing will help balance the left and right parts of the brain.
OPPOSITE: A beautiful place that's still, warm and comfortable will aid your meditation session.

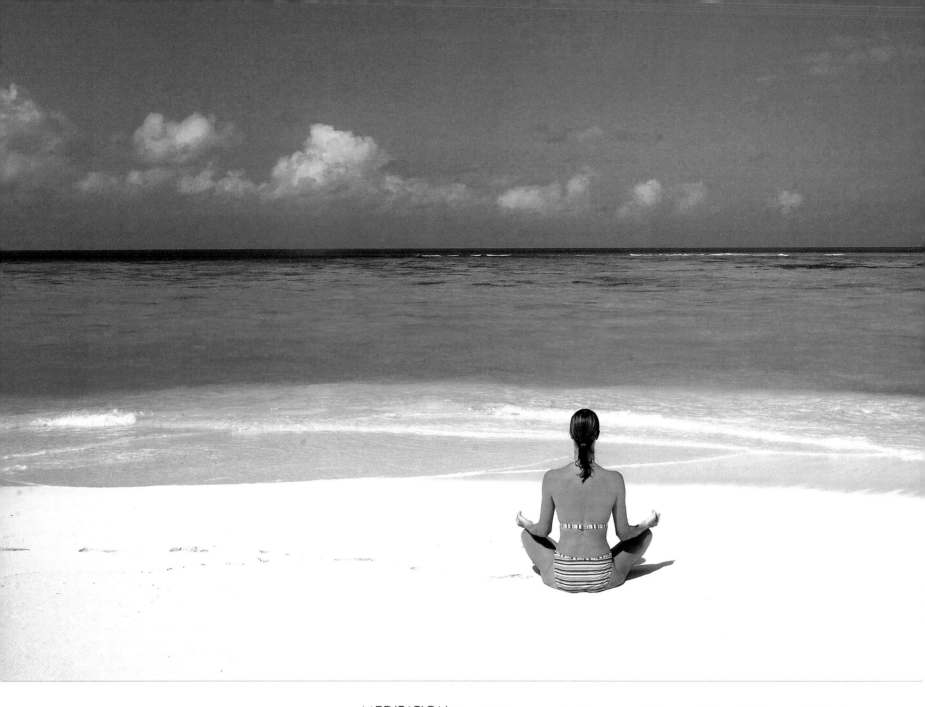

MEDITATION The mind is far more chaotic and active than the physical body could ever be. Considered by many as the highest form of yoga, meditation or *dhyana* calms and stills the mind like no other known practice. During meditation, the pulse slows, blood pressure drops and the brain relaxes, eliminating stress and providing a sense of real peace and tranquillity. And it is only when you start to really observe yourself in the moment that you realize the incessant nature of your thoughts.

Meditation provides relief from stress, offering the soul the space to live in the present. It has proven to be one of the most effective spiritual exercises and an absolute essential for attaining *samadhi* or ultimate enlightenment. The mind is powerful, but when it is full of thoughts there is little space for creative energy, so simply giving it a break allows nature to rebalance and revitalize. Scientific research has shown that those who practise regular deep relaxation and meditation have greater activity in the lobes of the brain that promote joy and serenity. This is also the area of the brain concerned with pleasure and pain-relieving hormones, like endorphins and serotonin, and may be one reason why practitioners feel radiant and more alert. Meditation, however, is no magical panacea. It involves the time and dedication needed to turn thoughts inwards and probe the questions of deeper levels of consciousness.

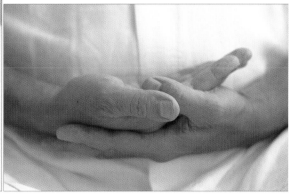

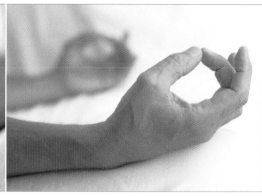

A JOURNEY FOR BEGINNERS Remember the technique is not critical, it is simply making the effort that counts. Do not force meditation longer than is comfortable and do not attempt to meditate after eating or when you are feeling tired. One very popular practice, that helps you focus, is to simply place awareness on the breath, following it as you breathe in and out and here's how best to do it:

- Find a quiet peaceful place where you are unlikely to be interrupted.
- Sit in a lotus, half lotus or cross-legged position on the floor (see page 133). Or, you can sit on a chair with feet firmly on the ground.
- Make sure you are comfortable. A cushion can be used if needed.

- The room can be quiet or, if preferred, some gentle, non-distracting music can be played in the background.
- Close your eyes and observe the flow of breath without trying to change it.
- Begin by taking deep breaths of equal proportion through the nostrils, always keeping the mouth closed. Count slowly as you inhale and extend your abdomen before exhaling slowly and completely through the nostrils.
- Hold the breath for a few seconds before both inhalation and exhalation.
- Once a comfortable rhythm is developed, you can stop counting—just follow the breath.
- If the mind wanders, gently bring it back to the breath. Sooner or later the inner world will calm.

FROM LEFT: The true lotus pose combines core strength with serenity, the latter doesn't come without the former; A meditation gesture where both hands rest on the lap, with the right hand on top of the left; Another gesture for peace and unity, where hands rest on the knees, with the thumb and finger lightly touching.

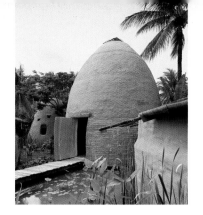

Meditation is a way of clearing the mental clutter that surrounds the subconscious. And when our minds are clear, we can see and experience the joy of our own soul.

-Gurmukh

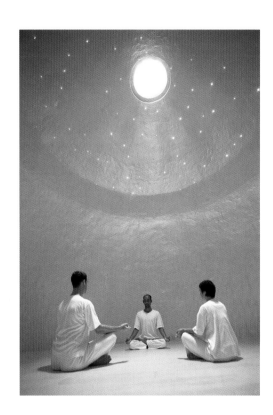

FROM TOP: The Earth Spa at Evason Hideaway, Hua Hin, with its circular domed huts made entirely of clay-like mud of mixed with rice husks and straw. The rooms remain cool even in the hottest of temperatures; Natural light infuses the meditation cave.
OPPOSITE: Finding a peaceful spot to meditate is key.

GETTING STARTED
To begin your spiritual growth, the most important consideration is finding some quiet space during a deafening day. To help, refer to the following guidelines:
• While you can meditate at any time, sunrise/early morning is best and you should always be facing the sun.
• Meditate regularly, at least once a day.
• Wash hands and face to freshen up before commencing.
• Outer harmony furthers inner balance and, although a beautiful calm setting is not essential it does help. If practising in the home, try to create a special and calm place in which to meditate.
• Begin by taking a few deep breaths and resolving to dedicate yourself to the meditation process.

• Start with about 5 minutes each day and gradually increase your meditation by 5 minutes each week. Once you find your rhythm it becomes increasingly easy to still the mind and stay focused.
• Never force meditation. In the rare instance that disturbing memories surface, you should stop immediately.

FOCUSING THE BREATH By concentrating on the breath we can focus on the flow and sound, or the phase of the breathing process we are in and where it is occurring. For example, during exhalation and the holding of breath following exhalation, concentration is directed to the abdomen. This ensures that the breath is deeper and helps avoid shallow breathing, therefore increasing the supply of oxygen to the brain. Also, when inhaling and holding the breath after inhalation, concentration is directed to the chest area. Simply observing this flow of breath—and focusing on areas of the body where you feel breath the most—helps quieten the mind, freeing it of incessant thoughts.

INTERNAL GAZING Another technique for maintaining concentration is internal gazing. Hold the eyes in a steady position with eyelids closed. Direct the eyes as if you are looking internally at the abdomen, the navel, the tip of the nose or to the point between the eyebrows—the third eye. Alternatively, hold an image before the eyes, such as the moon or the rising sun. Breathe and count the breaths as outlined above. Gazing as an exercise is not natural as normally the eyes move constantly, even when they are closed. With internal gazing, the eyes are focused on a fixed point while the other senses are able to rest.

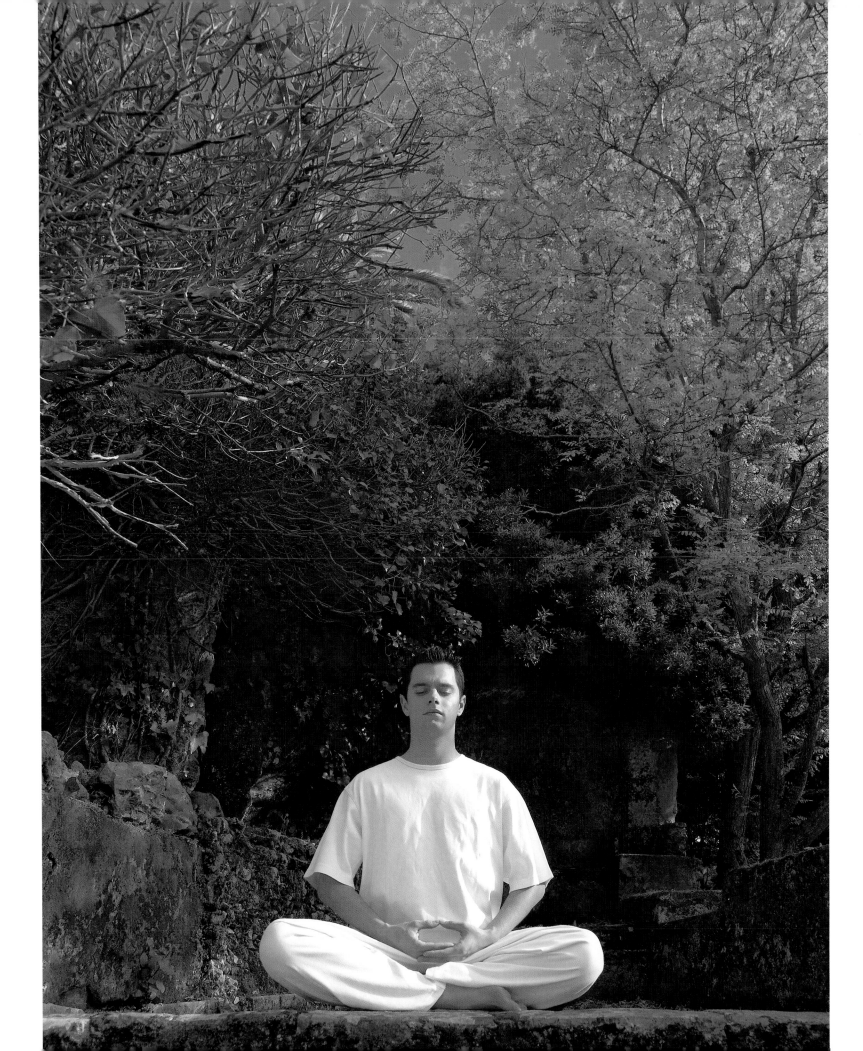

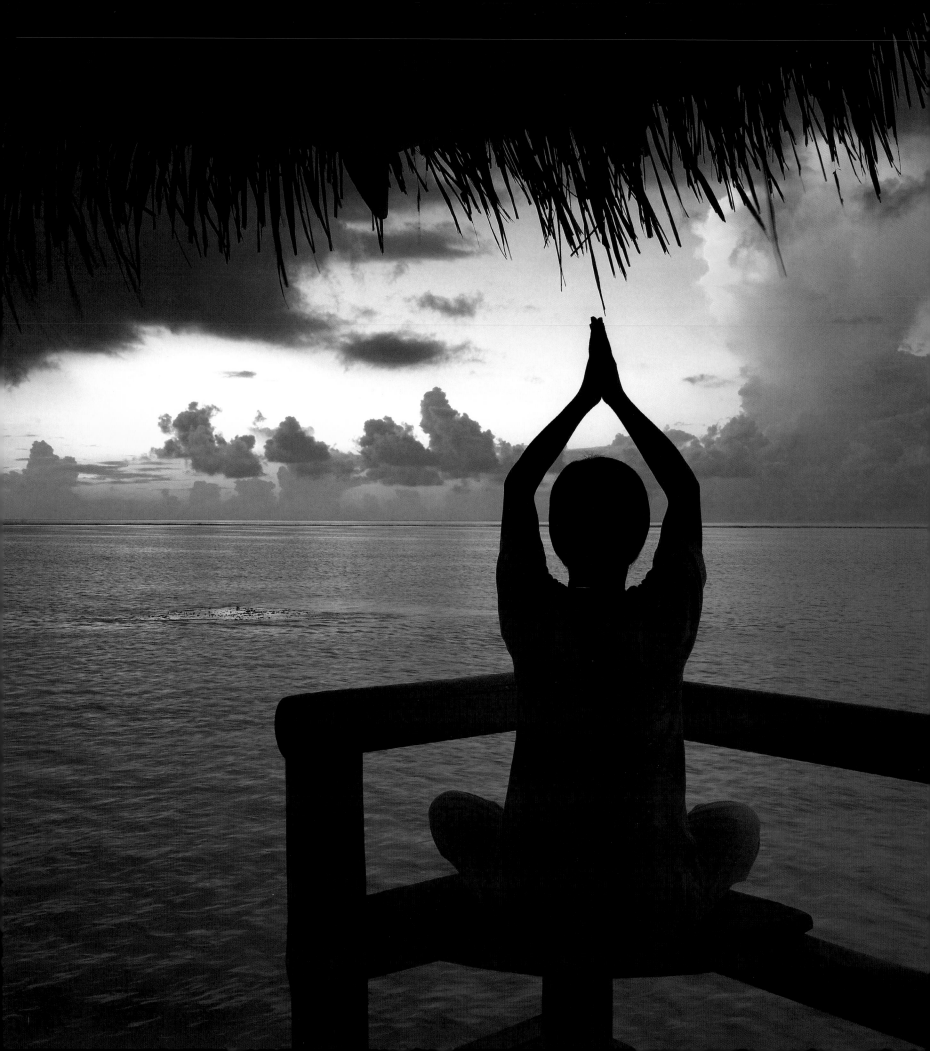

CHANTING Prayer is possibly the oldest form of devotion to someone who inspires spiritual dedication, and gurus worldwide recognize it as a powerful way of connecting with the spiritual self during meditation.

Sound is vibration and has the ability to alter consciousness, so one of the most widely used prayers in meditation is chanting. For example, a mantra, or Vedic hymn, is now widely used. Mantras are either spoken aloud or repeated mentally or silently during meditation. When sung it is called chanting.

One of the simplest and best-known mantras is *om*, the primordial sound in Sanskrit and considered to be the all-connecting sound of the universe. Chanting *om* is an excellent exercise for beginning any form of meditation as it helps bring the mind to a calm place from where the focus of meditation begins.

Chanting can be done alone, but in a group setting the effect is amplified and becomes even more powerful. The chanting may not flow easily at first, but it becomes remarkably easier with time as the voice becomes more confident and the practice becomes less intimidating.

THE LOTUS POSTURES

Although Confucianism, Buddhism and Taoism have handed down **96** different meditation postures, the most popular remains the Buddhist full or half lotus position of crossing the legs. Also called the seven branch sitting method, a correct lotus position involves seven key body positions. They are as follows:

- Cross both legs as below. If you cannot achieve this, then cross just one leg over the other in the half-lotus position.
- The head, neck and spine must remain straight at all times.
- Rest the right hand in the left hand, palms facing upwards, with tips of the thumbs touching. This is called the samadhi seal. Or rest hands on the knees with thumb and forefinger touching.
- Keep shoulders erect and free from tension. Do not let them fall forward.
- Straighten the head, pull back the chin.
- Open the eyes slightly—seeing without looking. Fix your sight about 2 m / 7–8 ft in front of you. In the beginning, you may find it easier to close the eyes to stop them from wandering.
- Put the tongue to the salivary gland of the top gums.

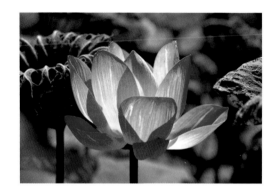

HOW TO CHANT

Repeat *om*, or a similar word, inwardly to yourself. Do not move the lips, just hear the sound in your mind. Repeat it over and over, several times during each breath, and let your thoughts come and pass without becoming involved with them. Once a rhythm is established, slow the repetitions, but speed up again if thoughts start to disturb the quietness. Slow down again once rhythm is restored.

You can also begin by chanting aloud for 5 minutes, whispering for 5 minutes and silently for 5 minutes. Then remain still focusing on the third or spiritual eye—the point between the eyebrows—and feel awareness expanding.

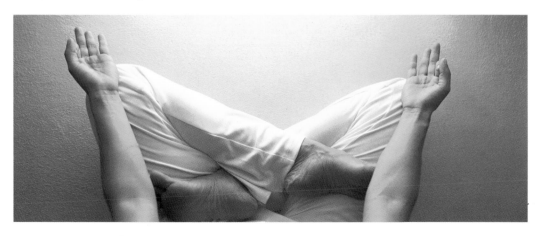

FROM TOP: The unfurling petals of the lotus flower symbolize deep meditation, where the layers of consciousness peel open in the mind and the body opens from a strong tranquil core; Dana-mudra, the gesture of giving.
OPPOSITE: Saluting the gods at Soneva Gili in the Maldives.

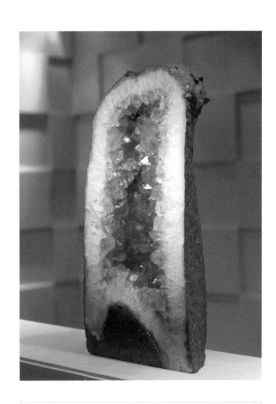

SPIRIT THERAPIES

Healing experts have long believed that we are more than the matter of our physical bodies; we have an energy body that vibrates at will each time we release a thought. Energy healing, also referred to as vibrational medicine, looks beyond the physical, viewing the human body as a network of complex energy fields that connect at the cellular level. Vibrational therapy targets these powerful energetic components that may be out of balance due to disease or disruption, and restores balance and order to the body.

CRYSTAL AND GEM THERAPY

Stones have been used for centuries for healing common ailments to bestowing status, luck and health on their owners. The ancient shamans used crystals in soul healing, as did the Australian Aboriginals who, in some cases, went so far as to sew crystals under the skin.

Crystals bridge the gap between science and magic; as silicon chips they are used to receive, store and transmit information in computers, radio and telecommunications. In exactly the same way, they are used in healing and meditation. Crystals respond to all kinds of vibrations from the environment and what makes crystal therapy so powerful is that each individual can tune into their own unique energy. They have extremely high and exact rates of vibration, which can be precisely manipulated and used to modify thoughts, emotions and the energy fields.

HOW IT WORKS Lying flat, specific crystals are placed at strategic chakra points around the body to unblock trapped energy and promote balance and harmony. Used correctly, it is a powerful tool and as the body starts to feel heavier, so do the crystals. The practitioner may hold the crystal in one hand resting the other on the affected part of the body while asking the person to visualize energy channelling through the crystal. Alternatively, the crystal may be placed on specific acupuncture points to facilitate interaction with innate electromagnetic energy, or the person might be given a crystal to wear as a bracelet or to place in their room.

Different crystals have different healing properties and practitioners learn to tap into the crystals' unique energy, thereby enhancing healing. Turquoise, for example, with its high copper content is an excellent conductor of energy and was widely used by the ancient Egyptians to treat cataracts and eye problems. It is also used to revitalize the blood and promote tissue regeneration in wound healing. Crystal therapy is often performed in conjunction with reiki and colour therapy. It may also be used in absent healing when a practitioner endeavours to form an intuitive link with someone not in the same physical space by projecting energies from the crystal to the person in need of healing. Visualization is key to success, as both the healer and recipient visualize balance and ease of flow. The healer becomes simply the channel for pure positive energy as stagnant energy melts away and new vitality fills the energy field.

It's said a crystal's life energy can be charged or discharged like a battery. Besides clearing new crystals before use, it is essential to clear them regularly to rid them of any jumbled energy they may retain. As clearing methods can differ and the energy of crystals is so powerful, it is advisable to seek advice from an established energy healer. Some of the

---

THE AURA

Practitioners who work with auras believe that all living things have an electromagnetic field, body of energy or aura that forms an oval shape around the body. Yale University's neuro-anatomist Professor Harold Saxton Burr was the first to measure this energy field in the 1930s, calling it the L-field or life field and many psychics or energy healers claim to perceive its emanations intuitively. Others use biofeedback sensors, computers and photographic devices to record and analyse these fields. A person's aura characteristics are believed to change with illness, moods or the environment and can be a reflection of their physical, psychological and spiritual well-being. Auras are thought to have seven layered bands reflecting different facets of personality corresponding in colour with each of the chakras or energy centres.

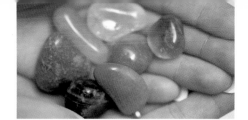

more commonly used crystal clearing methods include leaving crystals outside during a full moon, soaking them in a bowl of spring water with a pinch of sea salt, exposing them to the sun for 1 hour, or smudging them by wafting them with smoking herbs such as sage.

While gemstones are less evolved than crystals, experts believe that their virtue lies in their tints, their reflectivity and their energies, which will differ depending on whether the gem is polished, cut or in its natural state. For example, red stones like ruby and garnet relate to the base chakra and are used for calming and grounding the central nervous system. Another example: green stones such as emerald link with the heart chakra and are associated with love and understanding.

In the world of spa, crystals and gems are increasingly being used as vehicles for energy transfer in massage oils and specific therapies. Here, gems can be placed in bottles of massage oil blends, chosen due to their

harmony with the particular gemstone. The gem transfers its energy to the oil which, when massaged onto the skin, activates and rebalances the receiver's innate energy. Stones can also be placed on the body's chakras at the end of the massage to balance the body. When gems are used for healing they must first be purified by immersing them in salted water—or sacred waters like the Ganges in India—for at least 2 days.

CHAKRAS In the etheric body, the chakras represent a series of seven centres of electromagnetic energy located along the course of the spine. While they have no physical form, they directly influence specific glands and functions within the physical body. Each chakra vibrates at a different rate and has a particular colour and function assigned to it—see the chart below. For example, the base chakra, found at the base of the spine is ruby red in colour and is linked to the basic

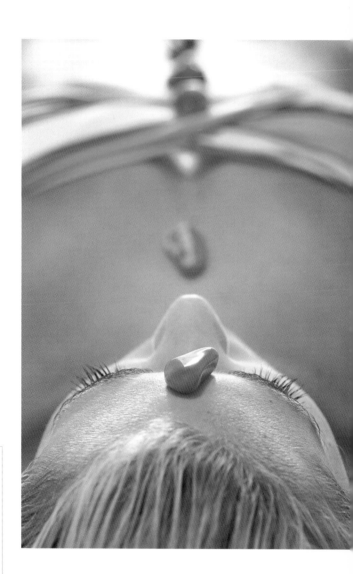

CHAKRA	Base	Belly/sacral	Solar plexus	Heart	Throat	3rd eye	Crown
LOCATION	base of the spine	just below the navel	mid abdomen	mid chest	throat	between the eyes	above top of the head
COLOUR	ruby red	warm and vibrant orange	bright and sunny yellow	emerald green or rose pink	bright blue	deep indigo blue	deep amethyst
STONE	garnet, ruby, onyx	hematite, moonstone	citrine, topaz	rose quartz	aquamarine	sapphire, amethyst	quartz, amethyst
GOVERNS	basic survival, connection to earth	sensuality and sexuality, guides feelings and emotions	self worth, stores and distributes basic energy throughout the body	love and compassion	self expression	insight and intuition	inspiration, enlightenment, cosmic consciousness

A selection of coloured gemstones; These gems are placed along the body's chakra points in order to relieve blockages and energize from within.
OPPOSITE: Unlocking blocked energy and reopening channels with crystal healing.

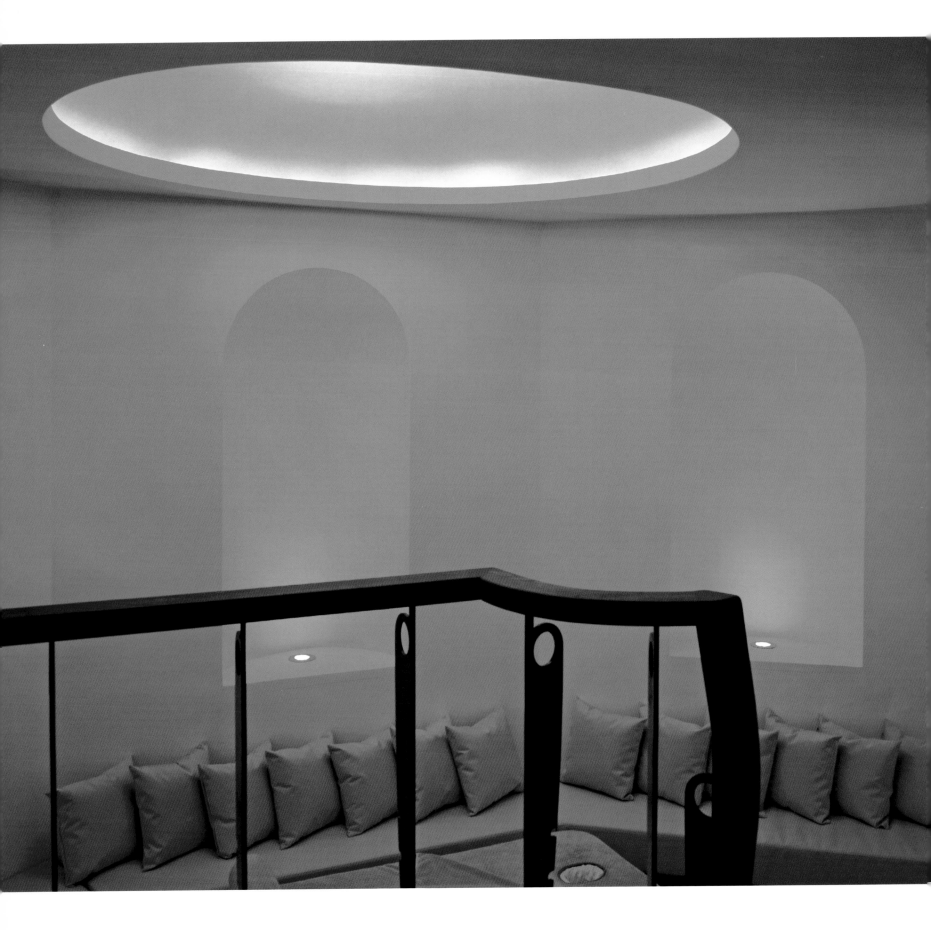

instincts of survival—think food, clothes, shelter and rest. Here, at the base of the spine, lies the *kundalini* energy, the sexual energy and basic instinct to procreate the human race. All chakras should be considered equally important and each must be kept clear and open to achieve inner peace and well-being. CHAKRA TUNING To tune into your chakra energy flow, sit in a chair with your back straight and feet flat on the ground. Close your eyes and start to feel the energy flowing in a spiral motion up from the ground through the feet and legs to the root chakra—at the base of the spine. Rest your attention here. Imagine the vivid red colour and see what comes to mind. This may hold clues as to the energy status of the chakra. Slowly spiral further up the spine to the sacral or navel chakra. Stop again and reflect on the vibrant orange colour before continuing your chakra journey up the spine to the crown above the head and slowly back again, through the centre of the body until energy is firmly grounded again through the feet. With practice, tuning into your chakras becomes far easier and is also an excellent way of focusing attention during meditation.

COLOUR THERAPY Colour is frequency of light that vibrates at different rates. We respond to colour, or light, instinctively and react to any lack of it. It's said that colour is a physical need that directly affects our emotional, mental and spiritual well-being and using these vibrations of light to heal is not new.

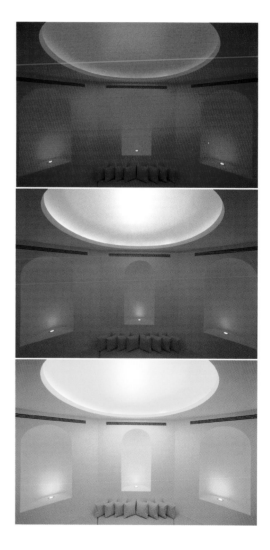

The healing power of colour, found in spas worldwide. Crystal healing is also commonly practised in a colour therapy room.

COLOUR ENERGY	GEMSTONE	HEALING QUALITIES
White light	diamond	balances the aura
	opal	energizes the chakras
Silver	moonstone	promotes inner growth (feminine energy)
Black	black tourmaline	energizes the base chakra
Red	ruby	represents stimulation and vitality yet grounding
Pink	rose quartz	represents love, feminine energy
	pink tourmaline	balances the heart
Gold	gold	represents wisdom, purity of spirit
Yellow	topaz	provides inspiration for the higher mind
	amber (yellow)	nourishes the nervous system
Green	emerald	energizes the body, balances the heart, and is a symbol of love
	jade	heals and balances the mind and body
Turquoise	turquoise	honours and protects the body
	aquamarine	represents clarity of vision
Blue	sapphire	aids purification and heals pain
	lapis lazuli	instils ideas and meditation
Indigo	blue topaz	provides creative energy
	fluorite	calms the nerves
Violet	amethyst	balances sexual polarity, connects with the cosmic world

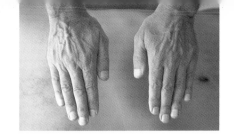

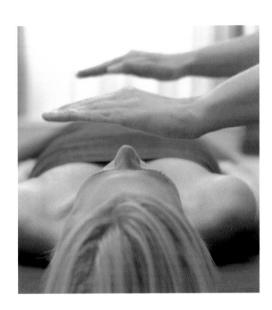

Just for today, do not worry.
Just for today, do not anger.
Honour your parents, teachers
and elders.
Earn your living honestly.
Show gratitude to everything.

-Dr Mikao Usui from *The Five Ethical Principles of Reiki*

Placing hands over or on
the abdomen during reiki is
believed to cure digestive
problems and relieve
menstrual cramps.
OPPOSITE: During reiki, hands
are placed at each side of
the head to help relieve
headaches and stress.

Indeed, the ancient Chinese, Tibetan and ayurvedic practitioners used the energetic aspects of colour to heal people on all levels, whether it be physical, emotional or spiritual or all three combined.

It's said that each colour emits its own subtle energy vibration that affects the body's chakras and associated gemstones. For example, red is warm, vital and heating. It loosens the body, releasing stiffness and constrictions. Red links with and stimulates the root chakra at the base of the spine, promoting the release of adrenaline from the adrenal glands and boosting energy levels. It is associated with passionate love, sex, impulse, action, strength, power and ambitious and temperamental people who have a need for personal freedom.

Blue—at the other end of the colour spectrum—is the opposite of red; it is cool and calming. Linked to the throat chakra, the colour blue governs the centre of speech, communication and self-expression. It is therefore associated with speaking your mind intelligently and with such qualities as honesty and integrity. For instance, a person described as 'true blue' means they are loyal and trustworthy. To make use of its healing properties, use blue when it is difficult to speak out, or you cannot find your voice. Try wearing blue when you are feeling anxious about speaking in public.

Methods of colour healing—aside from crystal and gem therapy—include the use of coloured light; try orange, which is great for socializing. Another method is the use of coloured water, for instance, taking a blue bath will help you relax and rest your mind after a busy day.

REIKI *Reiki* is a Japanese word meaning universal life force and is primarily perceived as a method of healing for body, mind and spirit. It is believed *reiki* was rediscovered in ancient Tibetan Sanskrit sutras during the late 1880s by Dr Mikao Usui, who went on to practise *reiki* in Japan, introducing it to other masters. Today, having spread around the world, it is one of the most extensively taught and practised spiritual and physical healing therapies in the West.

Reiki is an extremely calming form of touch therapy; the practitioner becomes the channel through which energy—or in Japanese, *ki*—flows to the client. This is done as the practitioner places his hands over or on the specific body parts that are in need of healing. The process generally starts with the head. When the practitioner channels this energy, or life force, through his hands it is believed to activate the client's own innate healing ability. This, in turn, rebalances the system as well as replenishes any depleted energy. For instance, placing a hand over or on the abdomen is believed to cure a digestive problem or ease menstrual cramps. While being credited with relieving a range of illnesses including arthritis, insomnia and migraine, *reiki* is also considered an effective form of self-healing.

Although *ki* is present in everyone, practitioners must be attuned to the ancient symbols before they can use *ki* to heal. This process of attunement is achieved in three stages or courses. The first course teaches how to work with *reiki* energy, the second teaches the three symbols that widen the *reiki* channel, and prepares students for mental healing. The third stage, the master course, initiates students where they learn a fourth, master level symbol as well as the ability to attune others.

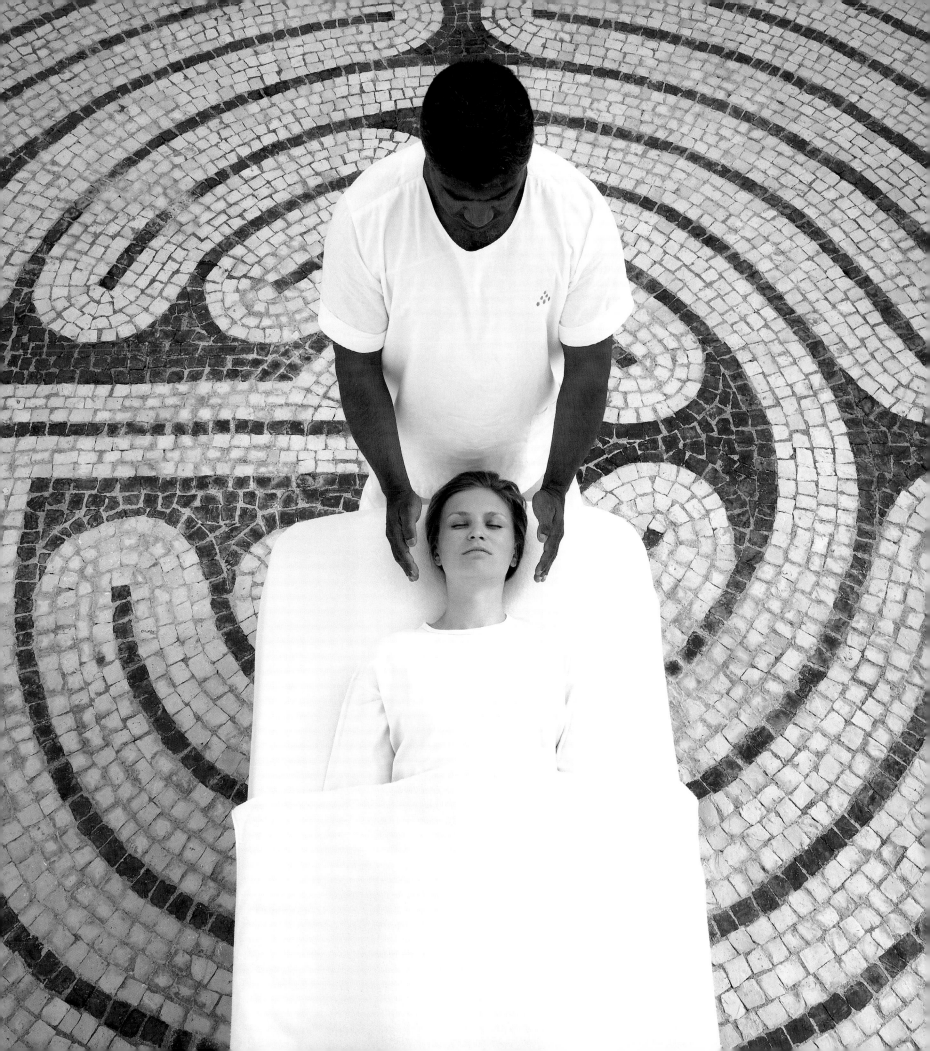

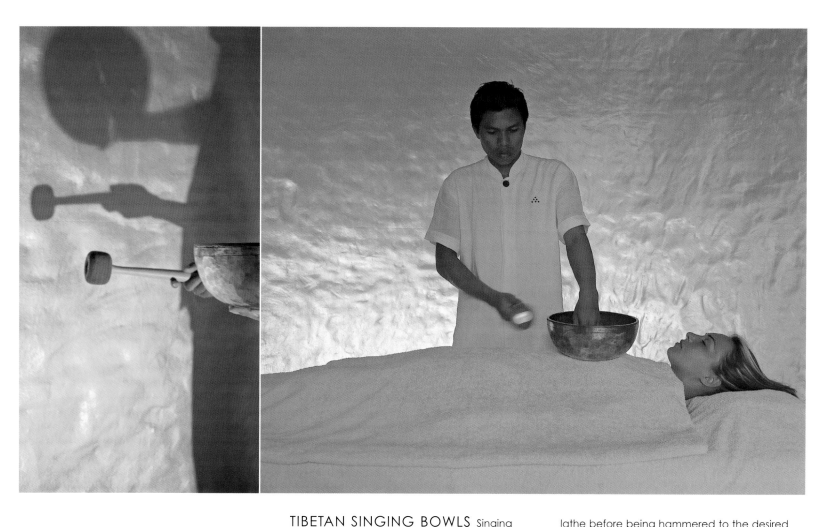

TIBETAN SINGING BOWLS

Singing bowls are believed to date back to the time of the Buddha Shakyamuni 560–480BC when the bowls were filled with barley, flower or rice water and butter. A thick wick was placed in the centre to create a butter lamp, which was then offered to the Buddha. In Tibet, the bowls were used for meditation and struck with a padded mallet or rubbed around the rim with a playing mallet to produce a fascinating blend of harmonic sounds that invoked a deep state of relaxation. The resonance and rich overtones of the Tibetan singing bowl are now common sounds in temples, monasteries and increasingly in spas worldwide.

Handcrafted by different makers, each bowl has a unique voice and magical aliveness that interacts in different ways with people and the environment in which they are played. They are made from an amalgam of up to seven metals and are hand turned on a lathe before being hammered to the desired hardness and pitch. Each metal used represents a different planetary influence:

- Gold: the Sun
- Silver: the Moon
- Mercury: Mercury
- Copper: Venus
- Iron: Mars
- Tin: Jupiter
- Lead: Saturn

HOW TO USE THE TIBETAN SINGING BOWL

Place the bowl in the open palm of one hand, or on the body part that needs attention, and hold the wooden stick or mallet vertically—like a pen—in the other. Gently tap the bowl and run the stick or mallet around the outer rim with steady pressure and speed. A series of calming tones will be heard. If not, try again until you hear it and you feel the body relaxing and starting to let go. Do not force the sound, it must come gently and naturally.

SOUND THERAPY

Sound is vibration. Sound is energy. Sound can affect our mood, health and lives. Some sounds soothe, while others energize. Singing bowls produce sounds in multiple octaves, invoking a state of deep relaxation which is believed to have healing and relaxing effects on the body and mind. The vibration is also believed to align the chakras and promote the free flow of energy through the body.

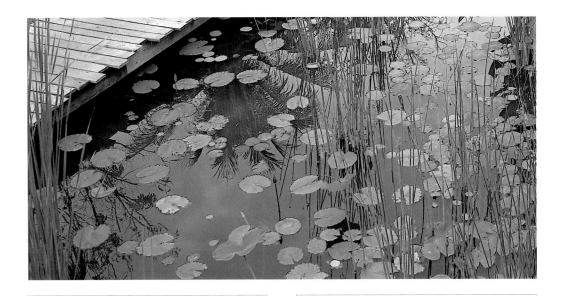

TIBETAN HEALING BREATH

This ancient breathing therapy helps rebalance the body, calm the nervous system and induce a state of tranquillity. Moreover, it's easy and can be done anywhere—all that is needed is a few moments and a comfortable position.

- Once seated comfortably, close the eyes.
- Turn the left palm upwards and connect the thumb and index finger to form a circle. Keep the other three fingers extended and straight.
- Place the right hand, palm flat, directly below the navel.
- Inhale through the nose. Follow the breath up through the nose and over the head. Continue down the spine until you reach the tailbone.
- Contract your buttocks.
- Release buttocks and slowly exhale from the mouth while pursing the lips together, like a whistle. Push the breath up the front of your body to expand the lungs and increase oxygen in the blood.
- Perform a second breath.
- Then move the right hand to the heart and anywhere else where pain or discomfort is experienced.
- Perform two more breaths, for a total of four inhale/exhale cycles and gradually increase the number of breaths.

This sequence of Tibetan breathing should be practised twice a day—early morning after waking and just before bed. It can be done while sitting, lying down or anytime an energy boost is required as long as you are in a comfortable position. If your throat gets dry, reduce the number of breaths.

JETI NETI

Jeti Neti or yoga's nasal douche is a nasal cleansing therapy that douches the nasal passages with a saline solution. By dislodging mucus it is an excellent way to clear blocked sinuses while at the same time clearing the eye passages and airways and improving overall circulation. A jeti neti vessel is similar to a small teapot, but has a longer spout to pour solution into the nostrils; see picture below.

- First dissolve 2 tsps of salt in 4 glasses of warm water.
- Fill the jeti neti pot with 2 glasses of the salted water.
- Tilt the head to the left and place the spout of the jeti neti vessel in the right nostril. The water should flow steadily through the right nostril and straight out of the left one. Remember to always breathe through the mouth to prevent the discomfort of water getting into the nasal passages.
- Refill the pot with the remaining salted water and repeat on the left nostril.
- To clear any residual water from the nostrils, a technique called a bellows breath or bhastrika should be used.
- While standing, put your hands on your hips. Bend forward until the torso is parallel to the floor, make sure the knees are slightly bent and not rigid. Keep the eyes open and mouth closed.
- Breathe deeply through the nostrils and relax the stomach. Breathe out with force pulling in the diaphragm. Do this continuously and quickly 25 times, turning the head right, left, and up and down for one breath in each direction. Then relax.

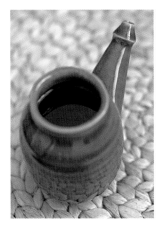

A jeti neti vessel, used for nasal cleansing, will clear blocked sinuses and open the nasal passages.
OPPOSITE: Tibetan singing bowls produce harmonic sounds that invoke a deep state of relaxation.

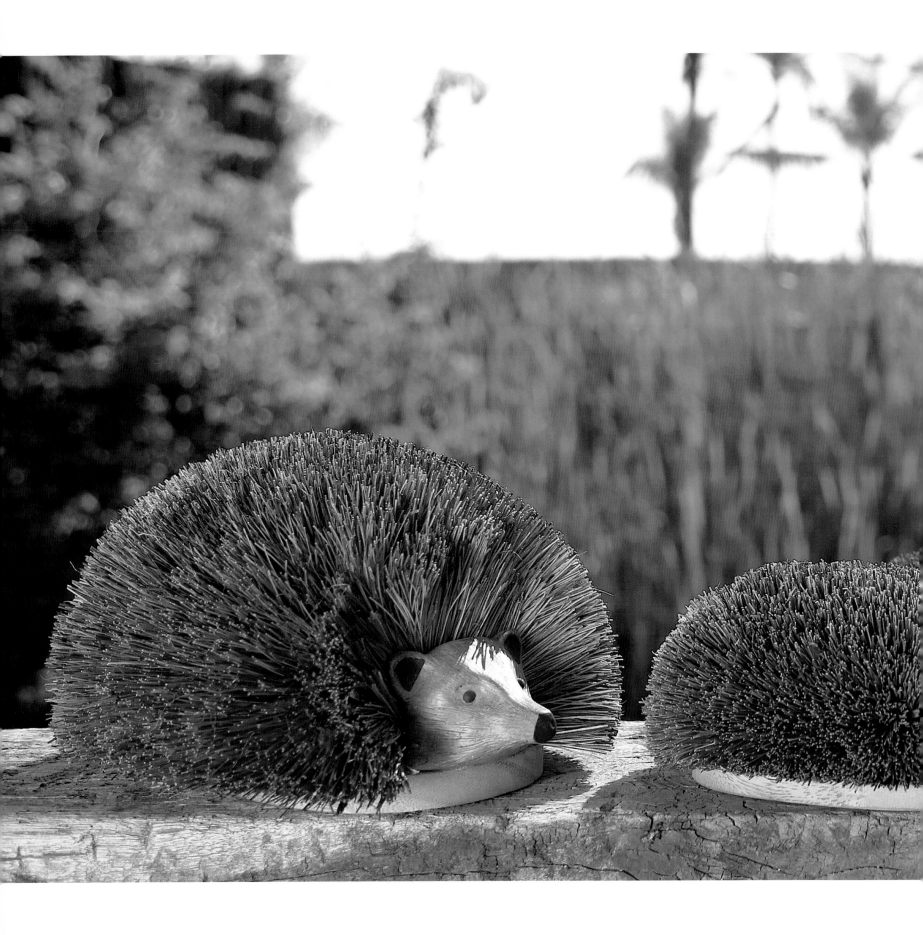

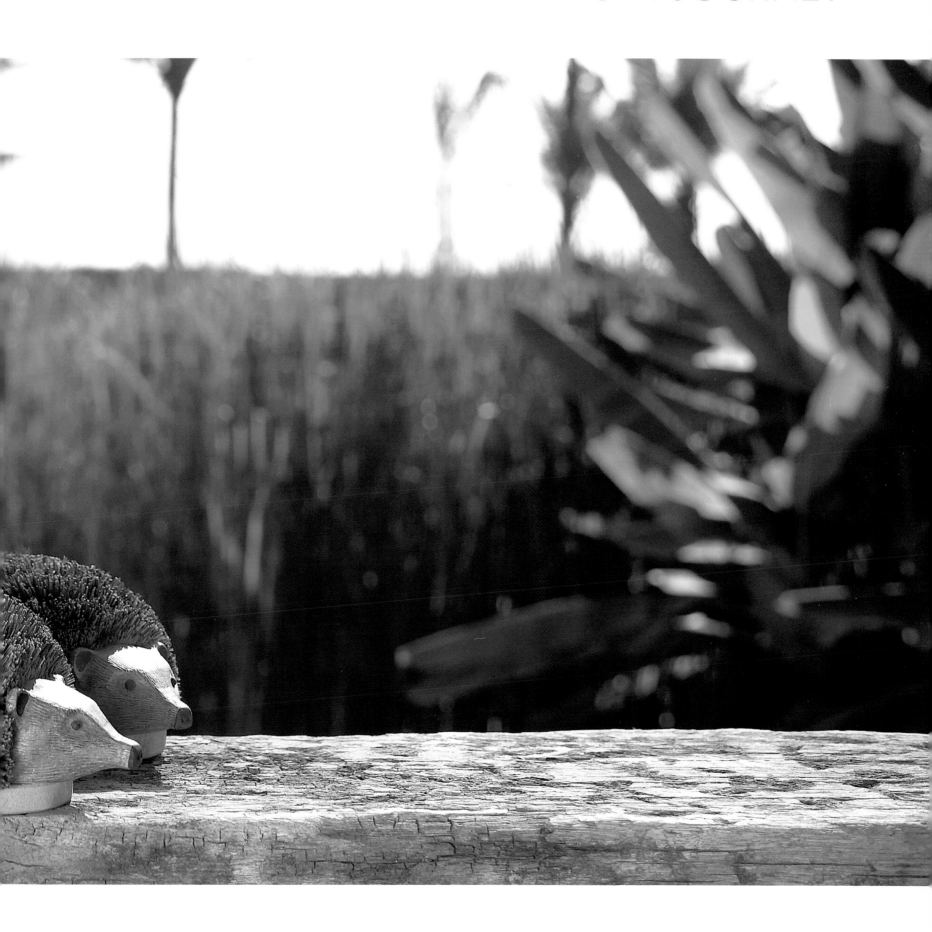

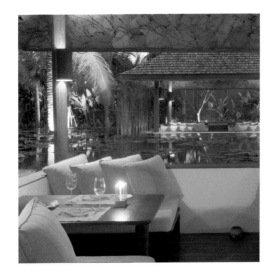

Rustic terra-cotta urns dot the grounds of Soneva Gili, and the cool water within is used to soothe bare feet that have been out for too long in the sun.
OPPOSITE: Over-water villas at Soneva Gili are constructed with natural materials, and come with novel touches such as a private sundeck.

SPA JOURNEY

It is the creation of experiences rather than a product that is at the heart of Six Senses' philosophy.

Founded in 1995, by husband-and-wife team Sonu and Eva Shivdasani, the Six Senses brands have become synonymous with luxurious living and cutting-edge concepts. Together the resorts present a refreshing reinterpretation of five star travel for today's more sophisticated spa-goer. Well-being combined with ethical responsibility for the world we live in, forms the central tenet to the Six Senses philosophy making them all leading and award-winning spas.

Soneva Resorts is committed to offering the highest standards of luxury in an environment that nurtures the area's indigenous feel in design, architecture and service. The resorts entail intelligent luxury at its best where nature fuses with an overall enchanting experience.

Evason Resorts offers redefining experiences that come hand in hand with contemporary and stylish design. Here, the emphasis is firmly placed on dedicated personal service for spirited experiences in desirable destinations.

Evason Hideaways is the boutique category of the Evason brand, where emphasis is placed very much on the attention to detail and on uncompromised standards of luxury. Elegantly designed and completely natural furnishings support the innovative style theme.

In each of the resorts, and integral to the core Six Senses approach, are Six Senses Spas. The spa's uniqueness lies in the quest for perfectly balancing the senses. The pyramid of six spheres used to identify Six Senses Spas represents the philosophy that is fundamental to the human experience. The pyramid's foundation consists of the three primary senses of sight, sound and touch. The second level satisfies the more acute senses of taste and smell, while the apex sphere symbolizes a sense of elation—the sixth sense—which is satisfied only by balancing the previous five senses. It is this, the unique experience of all senses heightened beyond expectation, that Six Senses aims to fulfil by instilling consistency and harmony between what is seen, touched, heard, smelt and experienced.

Six Senses Spas are designed as contemporary sanctuaries that adapt seamlessly to the host cultures and customs. So, wherever in the world you may be, you will be enveloped and nurtured in a truly authentic and ultimately luxurious fashion.

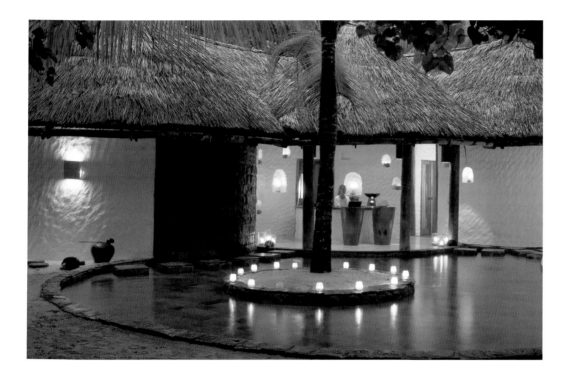

SONEVA FUSHI & SIX SENSES SPA, MALDIVES

Resting on its own private island, Soneva Fushi is the ultimate realization of the castaway fantasy. The incense scented Six Senses Spa is complete with waterfalls that trickle into the indoor pools, and therapy rooms that open onto a stunning lagoon. As flying fish dart past, guests are welcomed into what is undoubtedly the ultimate in soul therapy. Emphasis is placed on holistic therapies and many ingredients are grown in the organic vegetable garden before being moulded into nurturing recipes for the face and body. A refreshing range of traditional Maldivian therapies is available, the menu includes the Kurumbaa Kaashi Coconut Rub and the deeply exfoliating Veli Modun Sand Massage. Also available are Thai, Balinese and European treatments, as well as specialized ayurvedic programmes.

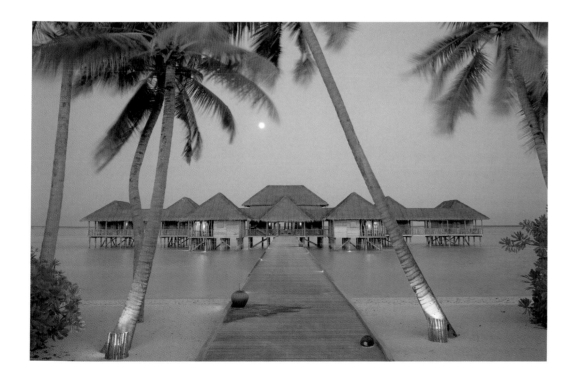

SONEVA GILI & SIX SENSES SPA, MALDIVES

Soneva Gili was the first all-over water resort in the Maldives with its 45 sumptuous suites and residences that are separated by wooden jetties. The cream of Maldivian resorts, Soneva Gili includes seven Robinson Crusoe Residences that sit on a private reserve and can only be reached by boat. The Six Senses Spa, overlooking the peaceful turquoise lagoon, boasts the very best of multi-cultural therapies from Hawaiian Temple bodywork, polarity therapy and ayurveda to the soul of Six Senses—The Soneva Gili Sensory Journey. During this signature treatment, two therapists work in harmony to treat the whole body, starting from the feet and ending at the face and head. With no less than five different stages, you are promised the ultimate journey of all five senses and beyond.

SIX SENSES SPA AT LE TELFAIR GOLF & SPA RESORT, MAURITIUS

Set in lush tropical gardens and surrounded by water, the essence of the Six Senses Spa at Le Telfair is a blend of time-honoured holistic therapies with contemporary cutting-edge treatments to cleanse and rejuvenate from top to toe. Two water encapsulated outdoor gazebos, each featuring a double mineral shower and oversized tub, are ideal for a romantic flower bath for two while the Honeymoon Spa suite—complete with couples therapy area, magnificent double bath and private pool—is the perfect place to experience the specialized blend of Aphrodite essential oils in the Couples Massage. Complete the experience with a flower bath and delicious fruit cocktails. There are saunas, Turkish hammams and six indoor therapy areas each with their own enchanting gardens.

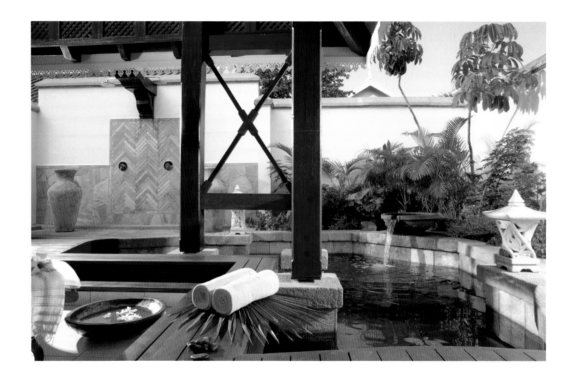

SIX SENSES SPA AT KANDALAMA HOTEL, SRI LANKA

Located in Dambula, 170 km (105 miles) from the capital Colombo, the eco-focused Kandalama Hotel rests serenely beside Kandy Lake, and is completely surrounded by pristine tropical jungle and flanked by two UNESCO world heritage sites: the Dambulla rock temple that dates back to 1BC, and the 5th-century Sigiriya rock fortress.

The Six Senses Spa is uniquely located on the hotel's roof and features six indoor therapy rooms, one of which is devoted to ayurvedic medicine. Each room comes with spectacular lake and mountain views. While the therapy menu is firmly grounded in indigenous ayurvedic healing, specialized body work including ear candling and hot stone therapy and the signature Six Senses Sensory Journey is also available.

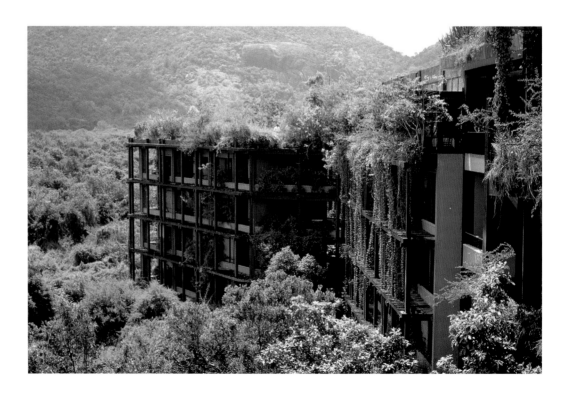

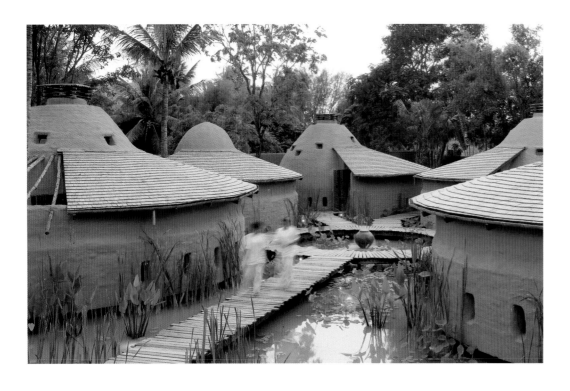

EVASON HIDEAWAY & SIX SENSES SPA AT HUA HIN, THAILAND

Adapted from a rural Thai village the Earth Spa at the Evason Hideaway is built entirely from a mixture of clay-like mud that's made from rice husks and straw. The mixture is then used to form circular domed buildings that remain cool, even in the hottest of temperatures. Inside these caves, the Six Senses therapists administer treatments. The coolest cave is reserved for meditation and is also the perfect spot for quietly cleansing the mind as it's bathed in the soothing sounds of Tibetan singing bowls. Emphasis at the Earth Spa is placed very much on skin foods with many of the ingredients being freshly picked for simple body-nourishing and feel-good therapies. Spa suites are also available, which come complete with a pool and massage champa.

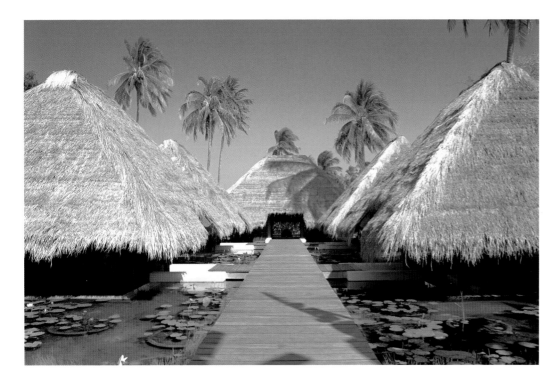

EVASON HUA HIN & SIX SENSES SPA, THAILAND

Nestled among 8 hectares (20 acres) of lush gardens facing the Gulf of Siam, Evason Hua Hin offers 185 luxurious rooms including 40 private pool villas. A totally new approach to materials, finishes and colours contributes to the fresh and unconventional design, and makes this a unique resort in Hua Hin.

The comprehensive menu of therapies at the Six Senses Spa is primarily based on natural skin foods that are freshly blended for rejuvenating facial treatments, massage oils, body scrubs and wraps. There is also a complete menu of wellness sessions featuring yoga in its many guises—such as ashtanga, flow, vinyasa and power yoga—pranayama, pilates and t'ai chi. Water t'ai chi is also available for those who need to loosen and nurture stressed bodies and souls.

SONEVA KIRI & SIX SENSES SPA, THAILAND

Situated on Koh Kood, along the east coast of Thailand, this spectacular self-contained resort comprises 46 luxuriously appointed pool villas overlooking the Gulf of Thailand. In true Six Senses style, Soneva Kiri is developed with the principles of ecologically sustainable design in mind, and construction methods are adapted so they protect the local environment. In addition to the many leisure facilities on offer, a highlight is the Six Senses Spa village with its all-inclusive menu of holistic treatments to soothe and uplift the body, mind and spirit.

Flights from Bangkok International Airport to Koh Chang take just 30 minutes by light plane. Soneva Kiri can only be reached by boat, so a speedboat will pick you up for the quick 2 km (1¼ mile) ride to the arrival jetty.

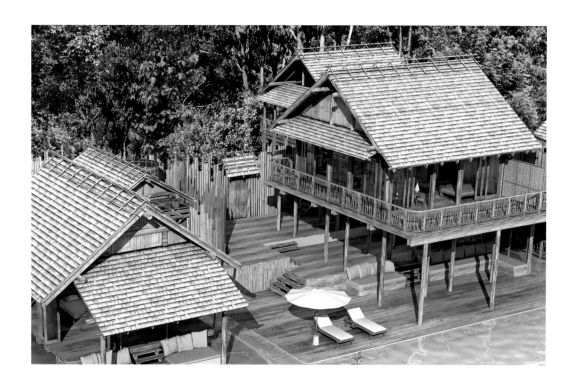

EVASON HIDEAWAY & SIX SENSES SPA AT YAO NOI, THAILAND

Sitting on the picturesque island of Koh Yao Noi, the Evason Hideaway & Six Senses Spa at Yao Noi is a 40-minute boat ride from Phuket, or just 20 minutes from Krabi. Comprising 56 pool villas in three unique styles plus a magnificent 3-bedroom Hilltop Reserve and 2-bedroom Retreat, all enjoy uninterrupted views over Phang Nga Bay.

True to Six Senses philosophy, commitment to the environment is paramount, creating an uncompromised standard of luxury with several restaurants and bars, a wine cellar and a chef's table. In addition to sailing, scuba-diving and rock climbing opportunities, the Six Senses Spa village offers a fully comprehensive range of face, body and spiritual therapies to soothe and uplift even the weariest of souls.

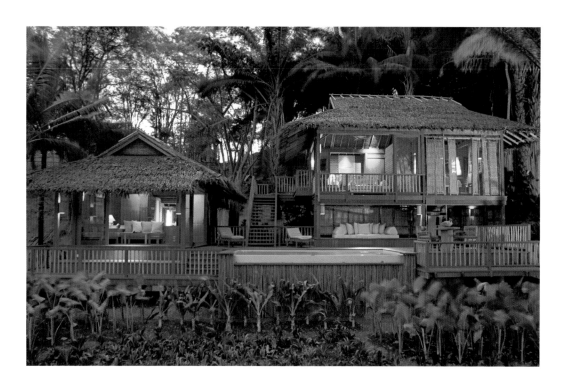

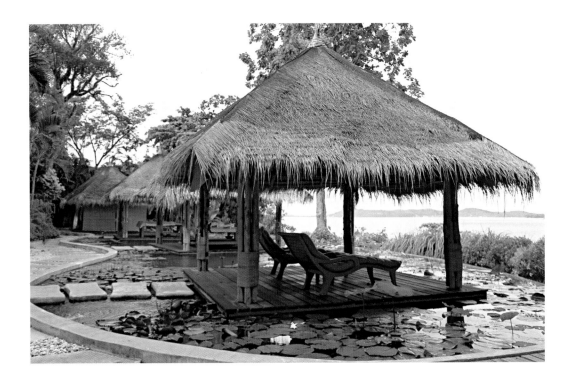

EVASON PHUKET & SIX SENSES SPA, THAILAND

An authentic castaway experience just 10 minutes from land, the fresh, contemporary and open feel of the Evason Phuket resort merges idyllically with the unspoilt environment. The luxuriously appointed Six Senses Spa spreads over three floors with double rooms and outdoor salas overlooking the Andaman Sea. A highlight of the inclusive menu of holistic treatments is traditional Thai healing therapies which include Thai massage and facials, Thai herbal compress, body scrubs and body masks and are all prepared with fresh local ingredients. For those who prefer a more international-style of therapy, there are rejuvenating face and body treatments and specialist body work including Hot Stone Therapy, Indian Head Massage, Hawaiian Temple Body Work, reflexology and reiki.

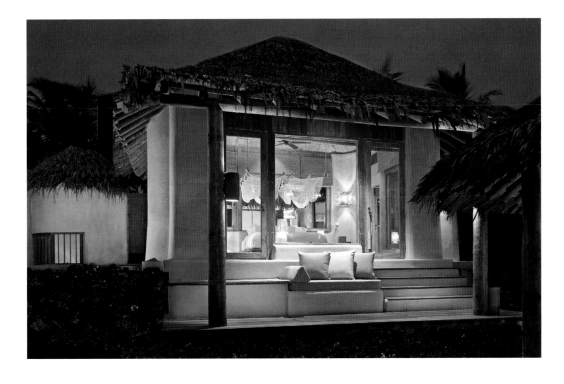

SIX SENSES ERAWAN— A DESTINATION SPA AT PHUKET, THAILAND

Located on Naka Island, just minutes from Phuket, Six Senses Erawan is the first Six Senses Destination Spa. Covering over 3,000 sq m (32,290 sq ft), the spa is designed to reflect an amalgam of Asian cultures from the varying indigenous locales. The Chinese area offers acupuncture, reflexology and t'ai chi with a very secret garden for sipping herbal teas. The arurvedic section has a yoga pavilion and verandah for authentic Indian head massage. Thai-style therapy features herbal steam rooms and a Thai Massage School. The Indonesian area, is for authentic therapies among waterfalls, outdoor showers and tubs. The fully comprehensive menu also includes colour therapy and a subterranean meditation cave for quietly cleansing the mind.

EVASON ANA MANDARA & SIX SENSES SPA, VIETNAM

Warm Vietnamese hospitality set in serene surrounds exemplifies the Evason Ana Mandara and Six Senses Spa. Setting new standards in spa design with natural tones mixed with traditional Vietnamese style, there are three sunken outdoor treatment salas surrounded by pools and miniature waterfalls. Traditional Vietnamese style salas, that are raised on stilts and surrounded by coconut trees, provide the perfect space for some relaxation or private consultation from the professional therapists.

Emphasis is placed on authentic healing experiences, and treatments include natural Vietnamese facials, Green Tea Scrubs and indigenous Fruit Body Smoothers as well as Vietnamese Flower and Herbal baths. All are complemented by Six Senses signature massages and holistic rejuvenation therapies.

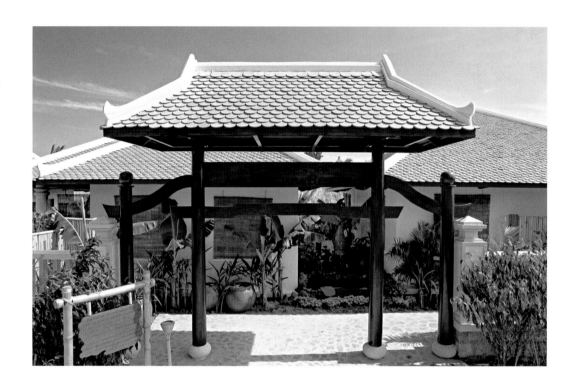

EVASON ANA MANDARA VILLAS & SIX SENSES SPA AT DALAT, VIETNAM

A luxuriously appointed facility, set within and around a French Colonial Villa, the stunning Six Senses Spa at Ana Mandara Villas comprises five therapy rooms, all with unequalled views across Dalat. The spa blends seamlessly with the unspoilt surrounds; for example, you can lie back and relax in an outdoor tub and enjoy the fragrance of the surrounding pine trees and organic flower garden. Here, the flowers are used to produce home-prepared essential oils for aromatherapy. Indeed, the spa focus is placed on fresh, natural and local ingredients that heal, pamper and rebalance the senses. The spa menu is an unrivalled range of indigenous and international therapies that soothe and uplift the body, mind and spirit.

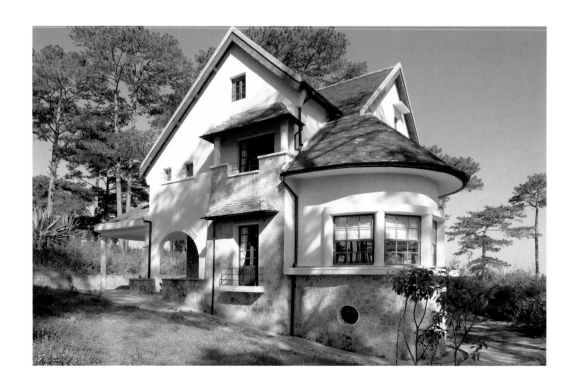

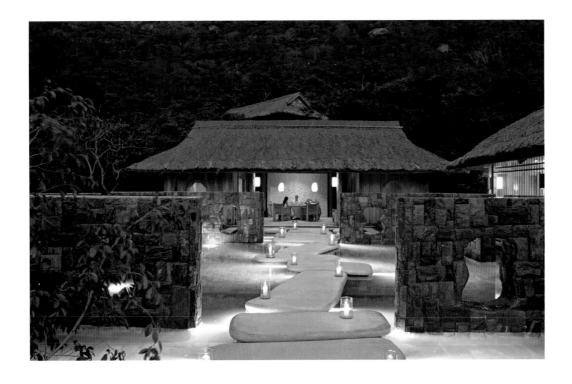

EVASON HIDEAWAY & SIX SENSES SPA AT ANA MANDARA, VIETNAM

Perched dramatically on Ninh Van Bay, overlooking the South China Sea, the Evason Hideaway at Ana Mandara merges beautifully alongside its pristine surrounds. Nestled beside a gentle waterfall, the open design of the Six Senses Spa allows the rhythm of the waters and the aroma of essential oils and incense infuse the tranquil space. On offer are some unique and naturally nourishing facial treatments and healing body therapies, which are all complemented with a range of authentic Vietnamese healing experiences. This is pure pampering in the hands of expertly trained therapists. The hilltop spa suites, complete with massage champas and outdoor steam showers, are a must for a truly personal and luxurious experience.

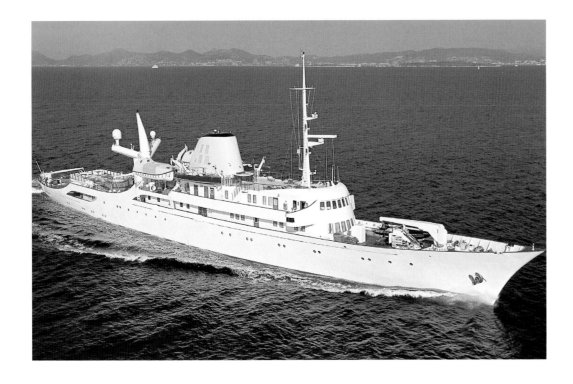

ABOARD THE CHRISTINA O

In yachting's rich and exotic history, little compares to Aristotle Onassis' legendary Christina O. Steeped in stories of visiting presidents, royalty and celebrities from around the world—each of whom has left their indelible mark—there is a mythical dimension to this super-yacht's complex character.

Like the Christina O, Six Senses Spa's mission is to deliver experiences that are truly unique and memorable. Using the very best in Asian and European therapies, which are delivered by expertly trained therapists, the Six Senses Spa on the Christina O is a haven of well-being and tranquillity that instantly soothes and uplifts. In Six Senses style, the spa adapts easily to its host cultures, whether it be the Mediterranean Sea, the Greek Islands, Turkey's Turquoise coast, Italy's picturesque coastline, or the French Riviera.

SIX SENSES SPA AT PENHA LONGA HOTEL & GOLF RESORT, PORTUGAL

As one of Europe's most historical estates, Penha Longa was once the summer retreat of the crowned heads of Portugal. The resort is now complete with two championship golf courses and a sumptuous 1,500-sq-m (16,150-sq-ft) Six Senses Spa. The spa comprises wet rooms, Jacuzzis, plunge pools, relaxation and meditation gazebos that are adjacent to the serene Jardin das Damas or Ladies Garden. In addition to the signature Six Senses skin and body therapies, menu highlights include the Golfer's Recovery ritual, that features a massage, facial and scalp therapy, and the ultimate four-hour Jardin das Damas Journey that treats guests to an exquisite rose radiance facial, signature body and scalp massage and hand and foot therapy.

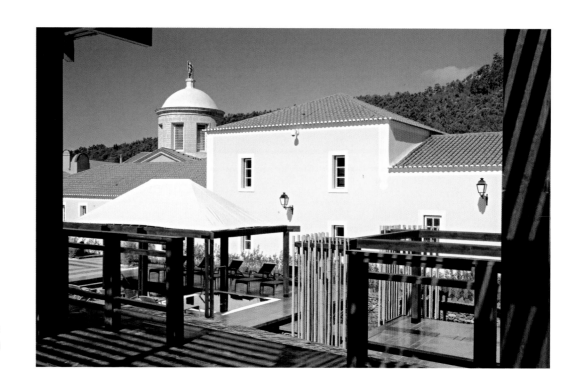

SIX SENSES SPA AT HOTEL ARTS BARCELONA, SPAIN

A sophisticated city spa experience in downtown Barcelona, the Six Senses Spa is perched on the 42nd and 43rd floors of this contemporary hotel. At such a height, the spa offers a stunning panorama of Barcelona as well as breathtaking Mediterranean views.

The comprehensive menu of treatments features the exclusive Hotel Arts: The Art of Stone Therapy and the signature three-hour Six Senses Sensory Journey. A totally modern spa, chromatherapy, which uses six individual colours to promote balance and healing in the mind and body, is incorporated in all treatment rooms and steam rooms. Also, there are separate ladies and gents wet areas complete with Klafs sauna, steam rooms, vitality pools and ice fountains that complete this modern spa experience.

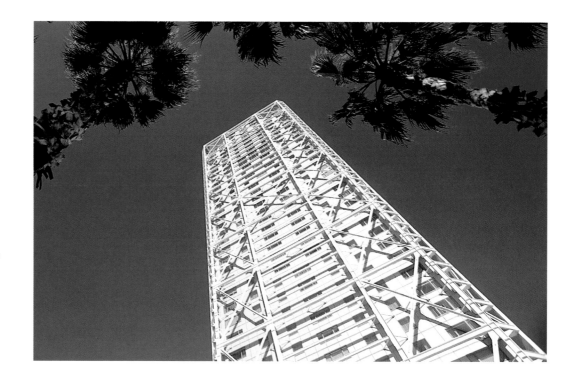

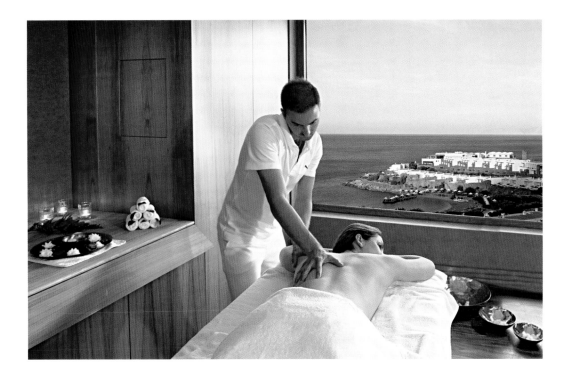

SIX SENSES SPA AT PORTO ELOUNDA, CRETE, GREECE

Located on a peninsula overlooking the stunning expanse of the Aegean Sea, the Six Senses Spa serves no less than three luxury resorts of Porto Elounda. Varying from hilltop hideaways to beachfront villas, this is the ultimate retreat. Featuring the signature subtle design of Six Senses, the spa is built on a gentle slope and the multi-level décor reflects the simple and discreet luxury that typifies the island's traditional style. While the all-encompassing spa menu goes beyond beauty and pampering to true healing, rejuvenation and the ultimate inner peace, a highlight is the authentic Turkish rose-coloured hammam, in which guests can enjoy some time-honoured and soul restoring rituals. Combined, the spa experience effectively appeals to all five senses, thus awakening the elusive sixth sense.

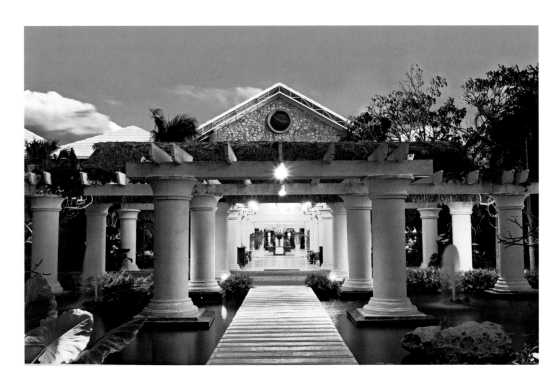

SIX SENSES SPA AT PUNTACANA RESORT & CLUB, DOMINICAN REPUBLIC

Eight kilometres (5 miles) of turquoise water, pristine white sandy beaches and golf courses highlight the extraordinary natural beauty of the Puntacana Resort & Club. Central to the Puntacana experience is the Six Senses Spa. Featuring the essence of Six Senses, the spa menu includes signature facial treatments, massages, hot stone and energy balancing therapies. Also on the extensive menu are Thai and Vietnamese-inspired treatments, harmonizing and revitalizing rituals, yoga, pilates, reiki and meditation. There are also uplifting signature journeys such as the Soul of Six Senses—a unique variant of the four hand massage that's administered along with a cleansing facial treatment and is performed by two therapists in perfect synergy.

SIX SENSES SPA AT MA'IN HOT SPRINGS, JORDAN

Just an hour's drive west of Jordan's capital city Amman, the healing benefits of the Ma'in hot springs and waterfalls have lured visitors for centuries. Legend has it that Herod the Great bathed in these medicinal waters. Now the thoroughly modern Six Senses spa houses ten treatment rooms, sauna and steam rooms all decorated in the Six Senses style. The spa sits directly over one of the hot springs that flows into the main pool.

Drawing upon local treatments and traditions, the spa menu focuses on the therapeutic properties of the mineral-rich waters of the nearby Dead Sea with salt scrubs and famed mud and seaweed wraps. The spa also incorporates a natural clinic focusing on enhancing blood circulation to the relief of bone, joint, back and muscular pain.

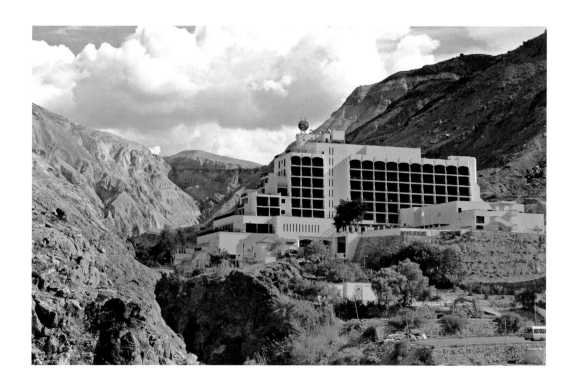

SIX SENSES SPA AT KEMPINSKI HOTEL BARBAROS BAY, BODRUM, TURKEY

The Six Senses Spa at Kempinski Hotel Barbaros Bay is designed as a contemporary sanctuary, it provides a taste of Six Senses innovative Asian heritage yet retains authentic Turkish spa traditions. The 16 therapy areas include three traditional Turkish hammams that are illuminated by classically styled columns on the pool deck, a chromatherapy (or colour therapy) room, couple treatment rooms, a unique private spa zone, eight personal spa suites, a purpose built watsu pool, high-tech gym and indoor pool and Jacuzzi. The healing and uplifting menu features the essence of Six Senses facial treatments, massages and stone therapies as well as indigenous hammam cleansing rituals and revitalizing journeys for the ultimate well-being of body and soul.

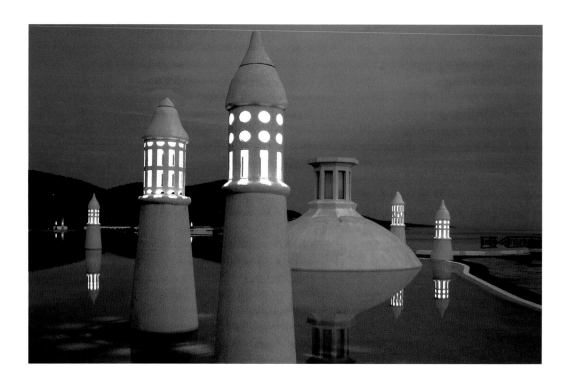

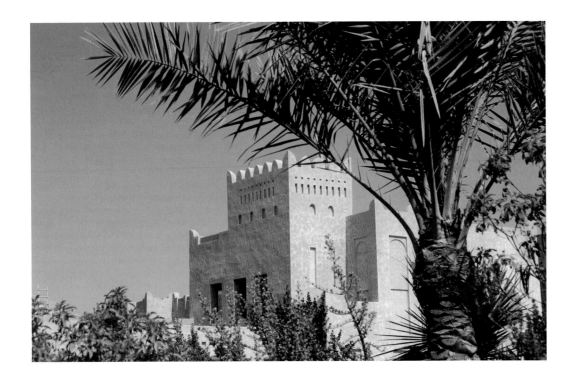

SIX SENSES SPA AT SHARQ VILLAGE & SPA, DOHA, QATAR

Reflecting a traditional Qatari environment the design of the Six Senses Spa Sharq Village & Spa, Doha is of a true Middle Eastern village with winding village streets, or corridors, and 23 treatment rooms resembling typical village houses. As well as the treatment rooms, the spa features saunas, steam rooms, Jacuzzis, plunge pools, and a fully equipped gym. A complete sanctuary, there are also dedicated yoga, meditation and t'ai chi, prayer and relaxation rooms. This vast yet tranquil space complements the spa menu, that's full of rejuvenating facial and massage therapies, scrubs, wraps and baths. The expertly trained therapists are on hand to deliver the best in service and therapy. Exclusively for women there is a dedicated entrance, relaxation area and beauty salon for hair, nails and henna treatments.

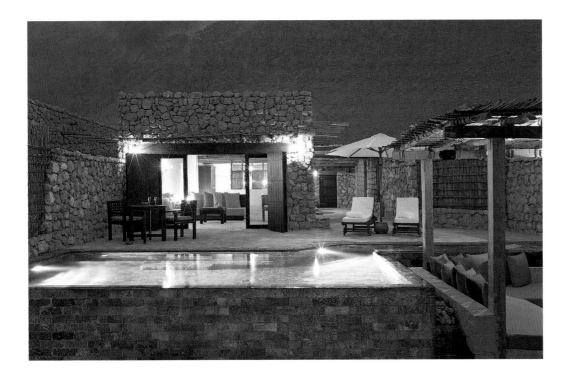

EVASON HIDEAWAY & SIX SENSES SPA AT ZIGHY BAY, OMAN

Set in a secluded fishing village in the Sultanate of Oman's northern Musandam Peninsula, enveloped by dramatic mountain views on one side and the pristine sands of Zighy Bay on the other, the Evason Hideaway & Six Senses Spa features 85 pool villas and pool villa suites, and a totally private marina.

In true innovative Six Senses style, a choice of dining alternatives is on offer, from a hilltop restaurant serving international cuisine to a central coffee shop specializing in regional specialities. A spa menu of unique and naturally nourishing facial treatments and healing body therapies, delivered by expertly trained therapists, comes guaranteed at the acclaimed Six Senses Spa with a highlight being the signature Four-Hands Sensory Journey.

SONEVA FUSHI & SIX SENSES SPA,
MALDIVES
Kunfunadhoo Island
Baa Atoll
REPUBLIC OF MALDIVES
Tel: +960.660 0304
Fax: +960.660 0374
Email: reservations-fushi@sonevaresorts.com

SONEVA GILI & SIX SENSES SPA,
MALDIVES
Lankanfushi Island
North Male' Atoll
REPUBLIC OF MALDIVES
Tel: +960.664 0304
Fax: +960.664 0305
Email: reservations-gili@sonevaresorts.com

SIX SENSES SPA AT LE TELFAIR GOLF
& SPA RESORT, MAURITIUS
Bel Ombre Estate
Bel Ombre
MAURITIUS
Tel: +230.601 5500
Fax: +230.601 5555
Email: info@letelfair.com

SIX SENSES SPA AT KANDALAMA
HOTEL, SRI LANKA
P.O. Box 11
Dambulla
SRI LANKA
Tel: +94.66.228 4100
Fax: +94.66.228 4109
Email: kandalama@sixsensesspas.com

EVASON HIDEAWAY & SIX SENSES
SPA AT HUA HIN, THAILAND
9/22 Moo 5 Paknampran Beach
Pranburi
Prachuap Khiri Khan 77220
THAILAND
Tel: +66.32.618 200
Fax: +66.32.618 201
Email: reservations-huahin@evasonhideaways.com

EVASON HUA HIN & SIX SENSES SPA,
THAILAND
9 Moo 3 Paknampran Beach
Pranburi
Prachuap Khiri Khan 77220
THAILAND
Tel: +66.32.635 111
Fax: +66.32.632 112
Email: reservations-huahin@evasonresorts.com

SONEVA KIRI & SIX SENSES SPA,
THAILAND
c/o Six Senses Resorts & Spas
19/F Two Pacific Place 1
42 Sukhumvit Road
Bangkok 10110
THAILAND
Tel: +66.26.319 777
Fax: +66.26.319 799
Email: mail@sixsenses.com

EVASON HIDEAWAY & SIX SENSES
SPA AT YAO NOI, THAILAND
55 Moo 5 Tambol Koh Yao Noi
Amphur Koh Yao
Phang-Nga 82160
THAILAND
Tel: +66.76.418 500
Email: reservations-yaonoi@evasonhideaways.com

EVASON PHUKET & SIX SENSES SPA,
THAILAND
100 Vised Road
Moo 2 Tambol Rawai
Muang District
Phuket 83100
THAILAND
Tel: +66.76.381 010
Fax: +66.76.381 018
Email: reservations-phuket@evasonresorts.com

SIX SENSES ERAWAN—
A DESTINATION SPA AT PHUKET,
THAILAND
c/o Six Senses Resorts & Spas
19/F Two Pacific Place Building
142 Sukhumvit Road
Klongtoey
Bangkok 10110
THAILAND
Tel: +66.26.319 777
Fax: +66.26.319 799
Email: mail@sixsenses.com

EVASON ANA MANDARA & SIX SENSES
SPA, VIETNAM
Beachside Tran Phu Boulevard
Nha Trang
Khanh Hoa Province
VIETNAM
Tel: +84.58.829 829
Fax: +84.58.829 629
Email: reservations-anamandara@evasonresorts.com

EVASON ANA MANDARA VILLAS &
SIX SENSES SPA AT DALAT, VIETNAM
Le Lai Street
Dalat City
Lam Dong Province
VIETNAM
Tel: +84.63.520 558
Fax: +84.63.520 557
Email: reservations-dalat@evasonresorts.com

EVASON HIDEAWAY & SIX SENSES
SPA AT ANA MANDARA, VIETNAM
Beachside Tran Phu Boulevard
Nha Trang
VIETNAM
Tel: +84.58.728 222
Fax: +84.58.728 223
Email: reservations-anamandara
        @evasonhideaways.com

ABOARD THE CHRISTINA O
c/o Six Senses Resorts & Spas
19/F Two Pacific Place Building
142 Sukhumvit Road
Klongtoey
Bangkok 10110
THAILAND
Tel: +66.26.319 777
Fax: +66.26.319 799
Email: christinao@sixsensesspas.com

SIX SENSES SPA AT PENHA LONGA
HOTEL & GOLF RESORT, PORTUGAL
Estrada da Lagoa Azul
Linhó
2714 - 511 Sintra
PORTUGAL
Tel: +351.21.924 9011
Fax: +351.21.924 9007
Email: penhalonga@sixsensesspas.com

SIX SENSES SPA AT HOTEL ARTS
BARCELONA, SPAIN
19–21 Marina
Barcelona
08005
SPAIN
Tel: +34.93.221 1000
Fax: +34.93.221 1070
Email: barcelona@sixsensesspas.com

SIX SENSES SPA AT ELOUNDA,
CRETE, GREECE

72053 Elounda
Crete
GREECE
Tel: +30.284.106 8000
Fax: +30.284.104 1889
Email: porto@elounda-sa.com

SIX SENSES SPA AT PUNTACANA
RESORT & CLUB, DOMINICAN
REPUBLIC

960 Abraham Lincoln Avenue
Santo Domingo
DOMINICAN REPUBLIC
Tel: +809.959 7772
Fax: +809.959 7773
Email: puntacana@sixsensesspas.com

SIX SENSES SPA AT MA'IN HOT
SPRINGS, JORDAN

1 Hammamat Ma'in
Zarka Valley 11117
Madaba
JORDAN
Tel: +962.5.324 5500
Fax: +962.5.324 5550
Email: mainhotsprings@sixsensesspas.com

SIX SENSES SPA AT KEMPINSKI HOTEL
BARBAROS BAY, BODRUM, TURKEY

Kizilagac Koyu
Gerenkuyu Mevkii Yaliciftlik
Bodrum 48400
TURKEY
Tel: +90.252.311 0303
Fax: +90.252.311 0300
Email: reservations.barbaros@kempinski.com

SIX SENSES SPA AT SHARQ VILLAGE
& SPA, DOHA, QATAR

c/o Six Senses Resorts & Spas
19/F Two Pacific Place
142 Sukhumvit Road
Bangkok 10110
THAILAND
Tel: +66.23.319 777
Fax: +66.23.319 799
Email: sharqvillage@sixsensesspas.com

EVASON HIDEAWAY & SIX SENSES
SPA AT ZIGHY BAY, OMAN

Zighy Bay
Musandam Peninsula
SULTANATE OF OMAN
Tel: +9716.544 1232
Fax: +9716.544 1232
Email: reservations-zighy@evasonhideaways.com

BIBLIOGRAPHY

Desikachar. T. K. V., *The Heart of Yoga: Developing a Personal Practice*, Inner Traditions, 1999

Godagama, Shantha, *The Handbook of Ayurveda*, Kyle Cathie, 2005

Lee, Ginger with Lim, Catherine Zita, O'Brien, Kate and Tan, Annette, *Spa Style Asia-Pacific*, Editions Didier
Millet, 2006

O'Brien, Kate and Sing, Troy, *Qi!: Chinese Secrets of Health, Beauty and Vitality*, Creative License, 2005

Turlington, Christy, *Living Yoga: Creating a Life Practice*, Hyperion, 2002

ACKNOWLEDGEMENTS

The publishers would like to thank all those who kindly allowed us to include them in photographs for this book,
and those who gave their generous assistance on location. Special thanks are due to the management and
hosts of Soneva Gili in the Maldives, Evason Hideaway at Hua Hin in Thailand, and Penha Longa Hotel and Golf
Resort in Portugal; and especially to the Six Senses Spa therapists in these locations.

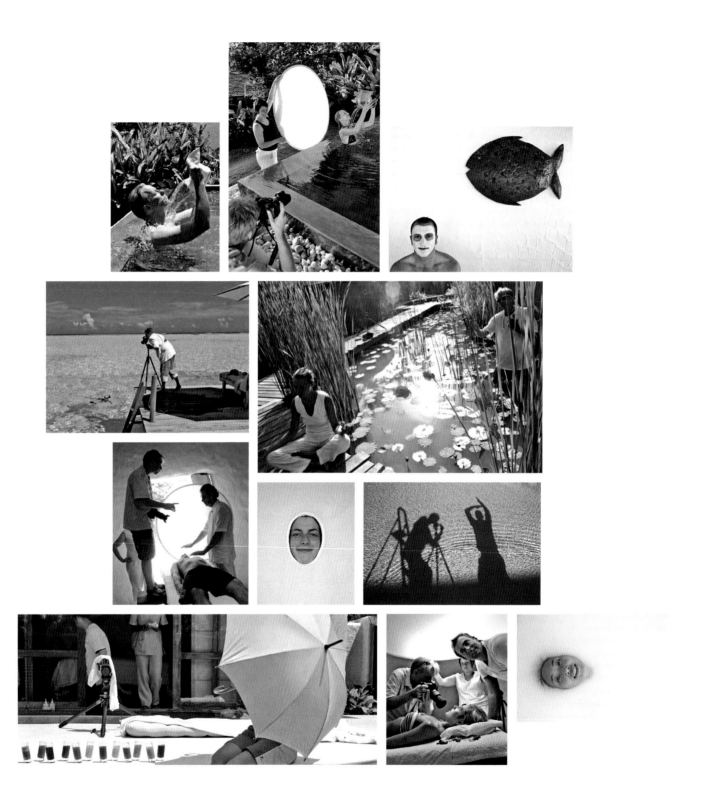

ADDITIONAL PHOTO CREDITS